W9-BYH-639

Dr. Bob Arnot's
REVOLUTIONARY WEIGHT
CONTROL PROGRAM

ROBERT
ARNOT, M.D.

LITTLE, BROWN AND COMPANY   Boston   New York   Toronto   London

Copyright © 1997 by Robert Arnot, M.D.

All rights reserved. No part of this book may be reproduced in any form or by any electronic or mechanical means, including information storage and retrieval systems, without permission in writing from the publisher, except by a reviewer who may quote brief passages in a review.

Originally published in hardcover by Little, Brown and Company, 1997
First Little, Brown paperback edition, 1998

Table: "A satiety index of common foods" by S.H.A. Holt et al. from *European Journal of Clinical Nutrition* 1995, 49: 657–690. Reprinted by permission of The Macmillan Press Limited.

Excerpts from glycemic index table adapted from "International Tables of Glycemic Index" by Kaye Foster Powell et al. from *American Journal of Clinical Nutrition* 1995, 62: 871S–893S. Reprinted by permission of The American Journal of Clinical Nutrition.

Excerpts from the "Eat More Index" from *Dr. Shintani's Eat More, Weigh Less™ Diet* by Terry Shintani, M.D., J.D., M.P.H. Reprinted by permission of the author.

Library of Congress Cataloging-in-Publication Data

Arnot, Robert Burns.
    Dr. Bob Arnot's revolutionary weight control program /
Robert Arnot.
        p.   cm.
    Includes index.
    ISBN 0-316-05172-1 (hc) 0-316-05167-5 (pb)
    1. Reducing diets.   2. Weight loss.   I. Title.
RM222.2.A754   1997
613.2'5—dc21   96-40190

10 9 8 7 6 5 4 3 2 1

MV-NY

Published simultaneously in Canada by Little, Brown & Company (Canada) Limited

Printed in the United States of America

Dr. Bob Arnot's

REVOLUTIONARY WEIGHT
CONTROL PROGRAM

ALSO BY ROBERT ARNOT, M.D.

The Best Medicine
Dr. Bob Arnot's Guide to Turning Back the Clock
The Breast Cancer Prevention Diet

WITH CHARLES GAINES

Sportselection
Sportstalent

To the millions of people
around the world
who suffer from the greatest plague
of our time,
OVERNUTRITION

Contents

Acknowledgments

My gratitude and admiration to Jill Werman, who through her skill, wisdom, and intelligence provided me with invaluable direction and research in writing *Revolutionary Weight Control*. Jill's contribution was exceptional and I thank her.

To my agents, Dan and Simon Green, whose perseverance and keen insight made this book.

To my editor, Bill Phillips, who offered creative suggestions and priceless counsel. Bill is the last of a breed of spectacular editors who make books far better than they might have been.

The following people and organizations from wide-ranging areas within medicine and nutrition took countless hours from their busy schedules to offer the most cutting-edge science in their fields. To them I offer my sincere gratitude for their enthusiasm, dedication, and hard work.

James W. Anderson, M.D., Belinda Smith, M.S., R.D., L.D., and the HCF Nutrition Research Foundation, Inc., who brought to light the vital importance of a high-fiber diet and first proved its amazing weight-control potential.

Stephen Bailey, Ph.D., whose anthropologic expertise added a great richness to this book and our understanding of how thousands of previous generations lived before us.

Luke Bucci, Ph.D., whose knowledge of the cutting edge in the field of nutrition assisted greatly.

T. Colin Campbell, Ph.D., Banoo Parpia, Ph.D., and the staff of the China-Cornell-Oxford Project, who provided me with their exceptional and fascinating research on nutrition and the peoples of China.

The staff at the Center for Science in the Public Interest, whose remarkable efforts to strive for the very best in consumer nutrition remains unmatched.

Bill Evans, Ph.D., who has consistently provided his research and knowledge in the everchanging field of sports science and nutrition.

Terry Shintani, M.D., J.D., M.P.H., whose unique work in bringing native cultural cuisine back to the Hawaiian people has transformed the way they view health care. Terry is a leader who, in time, will transform diets around the world.

Edward Horton, M.D., and the staff at the Joslin Diabetes Center, whose exceptional research on people with diabetes led the way for preventive measures for all people against the evils of excess glucose and insulin.

David Jenkins, M.D., who pioneered the unique and powerful concept of the Glycemic Index.

The staff at Native Seeds/SEARCH, who graciously invited me to their headquarters to see firsthand the wonders of traditional Native American cuisine and who invited me into their homes to eat the foods of our national heritage.

Annie Copps and the staff at Oldways Preservation & Trust in Boston, who introduced the concept of healthy ethnic cuisine through their outstanding work with cultures around the world.

Dean Ornish, M.D., whose well-known work in the field of nutritional intervention for cardiovascular disease has altered the way both patients and doctors view the treatment of the diseased heart.

Robert Pritikin and the staff at the Pritikin Longevity Center, who kindly accepted my request to learn more about their phenomenal nutrition program and who first proved that diet can be more powerful than medications in preventing and treating disease.

Margaret Wittenberg and Whole Foods Market, who have introduced this country to the first and largest whole foods chain of supermarkets, making good food available to the masses.

The staff at the Reebok Sports Club in New York City, who every day help me stay lean.

Walter Willett, M.D., Dr.P.H., whose extraordinary knowledge and keen sense of what really works has helped this project immensely. Walter has become the dean of American nutrition and is leading nutrition faster and further than at any time this century.

The staff at Canyon Ranch allowed me to visit their lovely Arizona location to experience how foods work as medicines.

- Jim Barnard, Ph.D., professor of both physiological science and medicine at UCLA Medical School and a consultant to the Pritikin Longevity Center, who first determined that diet could be more powerful than exercise in maintaining your health and weight.

I'd also like to thank the following for their keen insight, time, and breakthrough research:

- Michael Eades, M.D., a bariatric and family medicine physician in private practice in Little Rock, Arkansas, and coauthor with his wife, Mary Dan Eades, M.D., of *Protein Power*.
- Eric B. Rimm, Sc.D., assistant professor of epidemiology and nutrition at the Harvard School of Public Health.
- Elizabeth Lenart, Ph.D., project manager in the department of nutrition at the Harvard School of Public Health.
- Dianne Budd, M.D., assistant clinical professor of medicine at the University of California at San Francisco in the division of Women's Health Access.
- Redford Williams, M.D., director of the Behavioral Medicine Research Center in the department of psychiatry at Duke University and author of *Anger Kills*.
- Richard Wurtman, M.D., the Cecil H. Green distinguished professor of neuroscience and director of the Clinical Research Center at the Massachusetts Institute of Technology.
- Judith Wurtman, Ph.D., research scientist in the department of brain and cognitive sciences at the Massachusetts Institute of Technology.
- Michael Terman, Ph.D., director of the Winter Depression Program at Columbia-Presbyterian Medical Center in New York City.
- Michael Norden, M.D., author of *Beyond Prozac* and a practicing psychiatrist in Seattle, Washington.
- Richard Kogan, M.D., acting director of the Human Sexuality Program at New York Hospital–Cornell Medical Center.
- Raymond Lam, M.D., director of the Mood Disorders Clinic at the Vancouver Hospital and Health Sciences Center, and associate professor of psychiatry at the University of British Columbia in Vancouver.
- Woodrow Weiss, M.D., codirector of the Sleep Disorders Center at Harvard's Beth Israel Hospital and an associate professor at Harvard Medical School.
- Michael Devlin, M.D., a research psychiatrist at New York State Psychiatric Institute.

- Peter Jones, M.D., director of dietetics and human nutrition at McGill University in Montreal.
- Michael Jacobson, Ph.D., executive director of the Center for Science in the Public Interest and executive editor of *Nutrition Action Health Letter.*
- Jay Holder, M.D., D.C., Ph.D., the medical founder of Exodus Treatment Center in Miami, Florida, and president of the American College of Addictionology and Compulsive Disorders.
- Ernst Schaefer, M.D., director of the Lipid Metabolism Laboratory at Tufts University School of Medicine.
- Abhimanyu Garg, M.D., an associate professor of internal medicine at the University of Texas Southwestern Medical Center in Dallas.
- Scott Grundy, M.D., Ph.D., director of the Center for Human Nutrition at the University of Texas Southwestern Medical Center in Dallas.
- Jack Wilmore, Ph.D., professor of kinesiology and health education at the University of Texas at Austin.
- Ronald Kahn, M.D., director of the Elliot P. Joslin Research Laboratory and the Mary K. Iacocca professor of medicine at Harvard Medical School.
- Bill Evans, Ph.D., director of the Noll Physiologic Research Center at Pennsylvania State University.
- Angelo Tremblay, Ph.D., professor of nutrition and physiology at Laval University in Ste-Foy, Quebec.
- Robin Kanarek, Ph.D., professor of psychology and nutrition at Tufts University School of Nutrition and author of *Nutrition and Behavior.*
- Sarah Leibowitz, Ph.D., professor of behavioral neurobiology at Rockefeller University.
- John Fernstrom, Ph.D., professor of pharmacology and director of the Center of Nutrition at the University of Pittsburgh.
- Peter Jones, M.D., director of dietetics and human nutrition at McGill University in Montreal.
- James Stubbs, Ph.D., research scientist at the Rowett Research Institute in Aberdeen, Scotland.
- Jim Heffley, Ph.D., head of the Nutrition Counseling Service in Austin, Texas.
- Barry Sears, Ph.D., president of Surfactant Technologies, Inc., a biotech company specializing in drug delivery systems, and author of *The Zone.*

- Barbara Rolls, Ph.D., professor and Guthrie Chair in the department of nutrition at Pennsylvania State University.
- Paul Rozin, Ph.D., professor at the University of Pennsylvania.
- Bret Goodpaster, Ph.D., a postdoctorate fellow in endocrinology at the University of Pittsburgh Medical Center.
- Martin Marchello, Ph.D., professor of animal and range sciences at North Dakota State University.
- Arline D. Salbe, Ph.D., R.D., research nutritionist for the National Institutes of Health, National Institute of Diabetes and Digestive and Kidney Diseases, Clinical Diabetes and Nutrition Section in Phoenix, Arizona.
- Kenneth Blum, Ph.D., adjunct professor of behavioral sciences at the University of Texas Health Science Center of Public Health—Houston, and chairman and president of Kantroll, Inc.

Dr. Bob Arnot's

REVOLUTIONARY WEIGHT

CONTROL PROGRAM

Introduction

The principle of this book is simple: Foods are drugs. Choose the foods you eat with the care and love that a painter chooses his favorite brushes, and you will transform your life. How? You'll enhance your brain's mood chemistry to deliver the self-esteem, mental energy, vigor, and power to hold the line against foods that make you fat instead of depending on stubborn willpower to endure hunger. You'll fundamentally alter your body's physiology from weight gain to weight loss. You'll cut your hunger and craving for foods. You'll dump excess fat and gain muscle to reshape your body in the way you like. Do you doubt that foods alone really make such a difference? Remember that the high-starch, low-fat, low-fiber diet of the 1980s sent American waistlines sprawling faster and farther than at any time in history.

The primary stumbling block for most people to truly change the foods they eat is the unshakable belief that only bad foods make you feel really good. The core premise of perfect weight control is that the best foods will make you feel great *and* speed weight loss so that weight control becomes a joy, not a burden. You may trade in the short-lived hit of foods as recreational drugs, but in return you'll gain a day-long glow from the magic foods that have allowed people from different cultures around the world to lead long, healthy lives in perfect form. To change foods for a lifetime, you need only experience how much more terrific you feel and see the remarkable differences in your body.

There's little wonder we feel badly when we are overweight. Sure it ruins our self-image, and creates a stumbling block to social and business relationships, but it also consumes more and more of our time ruminating about it. The solace we often take is in the foods that will make us even fatter, robbing us of our self-respect. But there's another reason that we feel so bad: Obesity inexorably changes the way our bodies and brains actually function. We come to rely on foods as recreational drugs to attain fleetingly a pleasant state of mind.

The revolution in perfect weight control is that you can first control how you *feel* with foods so that you have the power to change how you look. Just think of it. If you felt great every day, you'd have no compunction about eating the right foods. It's the syndrome of poor eating — stress, anger, anxiety, fatigue, even outright depression — that drives us to eat the foods that will kill us. Yes! We're committing a slow suicide by using fattening foods to recover from the foul moods caused by eating badly in the first place, a classic catch-22. I call it symptom-driven eating. Here's what I mean: When you ask yourself the question "What do I feel like eating?" you're trying to make a diagnosis. You're asking yourself:

- "Am I fatigued?"
- "Do I feel fidgety?"
- "Have I lost my concentration?"
- "Do I need an energy boost?"
- "Did I let myself become too hungry?"
- "Should I reward myself for starving all day?"

If you answered yes to any of those questions, the chances are that your last meal played a big part in making you feel fatigued, fidgety, or anxious. Your last meal may also be driving you toward high-calorie, super-fattening "comfort" foods such as cinnamon rolls, French fries, or bagels with cream cheese as a cure. If you were a doctor, you would be up for malpractice: faulty diagnosis, botched treatment. In medicine, as soon as symptoms appear, disease has struck. The opportunity for prevention is lost. You now require strong medicines with all of their complications. When you cause symptoms by eating particular foods, you also create the need for strong food antidotes with all of their weight-gaining side effects. You'll literally need to eat a pound of cure when a few ounces of prevention would have done nicely.

This book will give you the satisfaction that you are finally bring-ing every major weapon to bear in the battle of the bulge. Perfect weight control will end your obsession with food and fat forever by giving you tremendous control over what you eat and when you eat it, to feel the best you've ever felt. You will gain mastery over hunger, compulsion, and fat so you can get on with your life. I've found per-sonally, as have many of my friends and colleagues, that our produc-tivity has soared as has success in our careers when we learn to take control of what we eat.

In the past fat loss was impossible to attain for most Americans without incredible dedication and personal sacrifice. In the dark ages of weight loss, tried and true methods were painful, had short-lived results, and were enormously difficult to stick with because they fought against the way the body naturally works far too hard. The long and short of it is that much of what was once used to lose weight was dead wrong.

WHY DIETS DON'T WORK

Despite thousands of highly profitable dieting centers, hundreds of bestselling diet books, and billions in low-fat food sales, the nation's most reputable obesity experts have declared an end to dieting! What! No more clock watching to the next rice cake? No more hypo-glycemic highs! No more rabbit meals? How did such a good thing come to such a quick end? How did dieting fail so miserably? Diet-ing has been declared the single largest failure in modern medicine, worse than many incurable cancers. Why?

Dieting is like holding your breath. You can only do it so long be-fore you have to say uncle. Then, like catching your breath, you're doomed to inhale nearly every scrap of food in sight. It is unnatural and perverted to diet. Losing fat hasn't failed as a concept, but dieting has. Eating smaller amounts of foods that leave you hungry and still make you fat is lunacy. Most overweight people find that as they eat less food they gain more weight because the wrong foods, even in small portions, powerfully signal their bodies to wrestle every last calorie into deep storage within fat cells. UCLA Professor Jim

Barnard, Ph.D., is struck by how obese patients eat so little of the wrong foods and still stay fat. Children in the 1990s consumed, on average, 20 percent less food than their slimmer counterparts did in the 1960s. From 1980 to 1991 the English decreased calorie intake 10 percent but the number of obese doubled. The great food paradox is that the very-low-fat foods that Americans turned to in order to become thin were the very foods that made them fattest.

What is lost in all the fuss is that there are millions of Americans and four billion people around the world who perfectly control their weight. Sure, we know everything there is to know about Oprah's diet failures. Like grade school times-table drills, every misstep is pounded into our brains over and over again, from talk shows to tabloids to talk radio. Failure is reinforced, whereas success goes unheralded, unobserved, and undisclosed. Eighty percent of the world's population has precisely the amount of fat on their bodies that they want, yet their secrets remain untold. In Central China, you'd be hard pressed to find anyone with a body fat higher than a marathoner. However, a superbly designed Cornell University study showed the following: Sedentary Chinese office workers weighed twenty pounds less than their carefully matched American counterparts even though they consumed 30 percent more calories. The difference between them and the rest of us is that they suffer no misery, hunger, or light-headedness. They feel great, look great, and yet still exercise perfect weight control, not through any magic of their own, but through foods passed down to them over the millennia . . . foods that have imbedded in them the ingredients that control their mood and their waistline.

A NEW ERA

At this point you may be saying to yourself: Where on earth did all these new ideas come from? It certainly doesn't sound like the stock-in-trade nutrition I'm used to. Here's why. Nutrition has moved from the backwater of science to the bleeding edge. Most advances don't come from nutritionists. They come from the leading fields of science in the world's premier scientific institutions.

Weight control is entering a new era. The fat-burning hormone, leptin, has been cloned. The brain receptor that kills hunger has been discovered by genetic sleuths. A new drug has hit the market which extends successful weight loss as long as ten years. The fat gene's magic weight-loss properties have been unraveled. New restaurants with superfoods are opening their doors. Engineered foods that control muscle development and fat loss are entering the marketplace. The medicinal effects of food are allowing researchers to plan meals that satisfy the brain as well as the stomach to cut craving, hunger, anxiety, even depression. The precise effects of foods on metabolism are being quickly deduced to manipulate weight loss. The habits, psychology, and physiology of success are carefully chronicled by the National Weight Control Registry. Yet most of us use myth, guesswork, and decades-old nutrition to control our weight. The good news is that there's a lot less willpower needed than you may think and a lot more smarts. This book unlocks the secrets of those individuals and cultures who successfully fight and win that battle every day. A generation ago, those "secrets" were largely bogus gimmicks, the backward practices of bariatric quacks who prescribed a medicine cabinet's worth of drugs, from amphetamines to thyroid hormone. Now, fat has gone legit. The world's top researchers lead the charge in the battle against obesity backed by the National Institutes of Health. Their results are published in *Nature* and *Science,* heralded on the front page of the *New York Times,* and reported on the evening news. Perfect weight control brings a remarkable set of new tools from their war chests.

I'm not a weight-loss specialist but I play one on TV, my friends suggest. As a journalist on the *CBS Evening News,* I have remarkably free-ranging access to comb the earth for the most exciting and interesting answers to the common problems that we face in late twentieth-century America, from the mountains of Nicaragua and northern Thailand to Japan and Central Africa. The ideas in this book aren't just theoretical science. They've worked for hundreds of people who've had an early look at perfect weight control, from my editor at Little, Brown, my producers at work, scientific colleagues, nearly

100,000 readers of *Turning Back the Clock,* to my wife, children, and friends. To be certain of its veracity I deliberately gained 18.5 pounds to test whether it worked easily and effectively. I put my career on the line. There wouldn't be many months left that network executives would put up with a fat, out-of-shape Dr. Bob. I'll share my own experience with you at the end of the book, rating what worked best for me and my family.

The Road Map

HOW TO USE THIS BOOK

The Big Picture: You will find at the beginning of most chapters a pair of high-concept slogans by which to remember the chapter. These slogans represent the conventional wisdom, and the new paradigm in weight loss, LEAN. As an example, in chapter 4, "Turn Off Hunger," you'll find the following:

Conventional Wisdom
An empty stomach makes you thin.

LEAN
A full stomach makes you thin.

After the big picture, there is a road map that gives you an overview of each chapter. Here's a brief road map for what you'll find in each section of the book.

PART ONE: THE STRATEGY

Rather than using willpower to cut down on calories, this section of the book makes foods work for you. Here you will experience a positive mental attitude and a feeling of fullness all day long while eating foods that can actually make you lean.

MAKE YOUR BRAIN FEEL GREAT

You'll learn how to use foods, supplements, devices, and prescription drugs to make your brain feel great all day every day so you have the mental wherewithal to shed fat. This chapter also details how the behavioral approach to getting thin has failed miserably. Diets cause terrible mental dysfunction — from depression to failed work performance — that parallels that of a person who has just had two stiff shots of vodka.

TURN OFF HUNGER

We overeat to make our brains and our stomachs feel good. Even if you've made your brain feel great, you may still be plagued by pit of the stomach hunger. This chapter has every great food to make you full and keep you full from dawn to bedtime.

DROP YOUR GLUCOSE LOAD

The biggest single threat to your waistline is the total load of sugars found in the carbohydrates you eat. This chapter lists all the most dangerous foods and the healing foods that cut the overload of sugar in your diet. By dropping your overall "glucose load" the very overweight can begin to shed pounds while those who are a mere 5 to 15 pounds overweight can at last kill that ring around the belly and those love handles.

PART TWO: THE ARSENAL

These are the most potent foods ever assembled for you to lose fat. The Arsenal rates foods for their ability to cut your hunger, drop your glucose load, and deliver nutritional strength.

HARD FOODS, HARD BODIES

This is the simple approach to weight loss. Eat hard foods and you cannot stay fat. Hard food is physically hard to digest either because it is hard to chew or slow to be broken apart and digested by your intestine. These foods kill your hunger, cut your glucose load, and turn off the hormones that make you fat.

PROTEIN

Protein is now considered the food of champions; not only for athletes but for anyone who wants to maintain the freshness of the early morning all day long and keep hunger at bay. This chapter has the leanest, most energizing, highest quality proteins for the mind and body.

HARD FIBERS

Fiber is the king of weight loss and perfect health. In this chapter you'll find out why. You'll also be able to pick and choose meals from a list of the world's most powerful fiber foods.

HARD BEANS

Beans are the dieter's true superfood. First cultivated in Southeast Asia as far back as 9750 B.C., beans give you a high-fiber, low-fat way of eating super-quality protein while killing hunger and cutting your glucose overload. The USDA rates beans up there with meat, poultry, fish, eggs, and nuts for their high protein value. Beans are called "gourmet preventive medicine" because of their wide-ranging effects on health, from breast and prostate cancer to weight loss and heart disease. In this chapter find out how the very best beans can work for you.

HARD GRAINS

Overhyped and outright dangerous in excess, most grains, quite frankly, make you fat. This chapter offers the grains that won't make you fat but will deliver protein, fiber, and a low glucose load.

BEANS AND GRAINS

Beans and grains are the only food combination on earth that gives you a complete nutritional meal. This unique and powerful combination excels at fat loss. It is a world away from the disease-promoting high-fat, low-fiber American diet.

HARD VEGGIES

Even though the world's healthiest cultures consume large amounts of vegetables, most Americans don't and won't. This chapter allows you to cherry-pick the most power-packed and effective veggies to keep you full and shed the fat. The best veggies for you are also the best tasting.

HARD FRUITS

Add the wrong fruit to the right diet and you'll pack on the pounds. Learn why in this chapter. Also discover the fruits which are most nutritious and still effective for weight control.

HARD FAST FOODS

From frequent fliers to long haul truckers, many people fail at weight control because their lifestyles don't allow them to prepare the foods that will work for them. This chapter is packed with terrific hard foods to eat on the fly.

PART THREE: THE PLAN

The Plan pulls all the fat-loss concepts in the book together to offer you a delicious, exciting, and effective way of eating in your everyday life.

FEEDFORWARD EATING

This is the payoff. As important as the actual foods themselves is the timing of their ingestion. More alerting foods in the morning, more calming foods in the afternoon, and more soporific foods in the evening. "Lose Weight Overnight" is not a tabloid headline. You can make it happen with the correct timing of the foods you eat. By learning to anticipate the druglike effects of foods in specific time "zones" throughout the day and learning to eat accordingly, you can feel, act, and perform exactly as you choose.

HARD CUISINE

Real meals that promote weight loss from the world's healthiest cultures.

PART FOUR: FAT-LOSS ACCELERATORS

To push the power of foods over the brink, these chapters will give you every last tool to promote perfect weight control.

FAT-RIPPING EXERCISES

Most exercise is a waste of time when it comes to its ability to rip off the fat. Fat-ripping exercises burn the maximum number of the right kinds of calories to make you trim and keep you trim.

BUILDING A BIGGER ENGINE

To burn calories at rest, you need a big, lean, calorie-burning machine. This chapter gives you simple, super-efficient exercises to increase fat burning twenty-four hours a day. These are the same excellent weight-training exercises recommended so strongly in the book *Protein Power*, by Doctors Michael and Mary Dan Eades.

PART FIVE: PERFECT WEIGHT CONTROL

THE GLUCOSE EPIDEMIC

There is one diet and one diet alone that is responsible for a scourge of food-borne disease that rages across the globe: the low-fiber, high-fat, high-glucose Western diet. Although fats were long blamed for the rising worldwide tide of obesity, it is the total amount of glucose released from foods into your bloodstream that is most accountable. By 2035, 100 percent of Americans will be seriously overweight if the glucose epidemic continues unabated.

TRUE CONFESSIONS

I've tried the program, I've lost the weight. Here's how it worked for my family, colleagues, friends, and myself.

POSTSCRIPT

THE APPENDIX

This lists all supplements and devices and where they can be purchased. (Neither the author of this book nor the publisher has any financial interest in any of these products nor do they derive any profits or concessions from them.)

THE GLOSSARY

There are very few technical terms in this book, insulin, glucose, and serotonin being the most important. If at any point in the book you find an unfamiliar term or want to remind yourself of its meaning, turn to the Glossary for an explanation. This will give you the confidence that you never need stumble because of unfamiliar terminology.

RATING

Not every measure in this book is equally powerful. For this reason you will find various measures rated using the following system:

***** Highly recommended, works like a charm
**** Highly recommended
*** Works well
** Worth trying
* Works, but not much noticeable benefit

WHO THIS BOOK IS FOR

This book delivers an exquisite and precise means of weight control. With small tolerances for calorie error, women will appreciate how perfect weight control puts them exactly where they want while enhancing their mood, avoiding dysphoria or malaise and the carbo craving that comes with PMS. It meets the demands of the most exacting and experienced dieting aficionado with fresh, unique, and fascinating material. Men who have not appreciated the demands that women have met for years to look exactly as they wish will appreciate how quickly they too can lose the bulk of their fat. Like women, they will discover that perfect weight control allows them to lose the last five critical pounds and gives them the cut look and shape of a teenager.

Foods as Drugs

Foods as drugs? Sound preposterous? You may think this is simply a metaphor. It is not. The *New York Times* called foods the pharmacy of the 1990s. At the Massachusetts Institute of Technology, doctors alter the mood of depressed and overweight patients with foods. Top Olympic athletes and the nation's armed forces use varying mixtures of protein, choline, and carbohydrates to enhance performance. Fighter pilots take the amino acid tyrosine to improve vigilance. Researchers treat food addiction with handpicked amino acids. Men cut their risk of heart disease 40 percent with 30 grams of fiber a day, according to the Harvard School of Public Health. Neurologists use a form of choline to treat strokes. Researchers are using soy protein powder to prevent the recurrence of breast and prostate cancer. Doctors even open up clogged arteries with plant-based foods.

For effective weight control, food is the most powerful and effective drug there is. If someone devised foods to make you thin, they'd be awarded a Nobel Prize for inventing a totally side effect–free, drug-free means of controlling obesity. But because lean, hard foods are so widely available we simply ignore them and wait, longing for a magic bullet to make our fat go away.

Conventional Wisdom

Foods are recreational drugs.

LEAN

Foods are therapeutic medicines.

ROAD MAP

This chapter introduces the concept of foods as powerful drugs that make you lean. The chapters in "The Arsenal" section give you a detailed explanation of how individual foods work to control your weight perfectly.

FOODS AS DRUGS

Each time you put a piece of food in your mouth, you are giving your body a very powerful set of highly specific instructions. Foods go to work far faster and with far more profound effects on your body than most drugs. For example, you must wait several weeks for the antidepressant Prozac to build up enough of the neurotransmitter serotonin in your brain for your depression to lift, but you can build large levels of serotonin in your brain in just minutes by ingesting carbohydrates. You might ask, Well, why don't depressed people eat lots of carbos for their depression? Many do! And grow fatter and fatter trying to make themselves feel happy . . . the wrong way. As an example, several large cinnamon rolls, liberally covered with frosting, can make you feel euphoric within minutes, but just as quickly a fusillade of fat-carrying particles are launched toward your waistline.

Ten years from now you will be able to manipulate your appetite and weight easily with genetically engineered drugs based on newly discovered hormones such as leptin, MCH, and Neuropeptide Y. But if you're hoping to control your weight in this century, consider that foods trigger the release of the body's most powerful fat-loss hormones and block the actions of potent weight-gaining hormones. I'll show you how to achieve those twenty-first-century results today with foods as drugs.

GEAR YOUR BODY TO WEIGHT LOSS

With the right foods you can change your body from a fat-sucking behemoth to a taut, lithe calorie-burning machine. Scientifically we say that you are changing from the physiology of weight gain to the physiology of weight loss. Curiously, during most diets, the physiology of weight gain cranks into high gear, so that the second your diet ends or you begin to stumble, you'll balloon again. However, once you change foods, your physiology will be transformed so that weight control is easy and sustained weight gain hard.

First let's return to the idea of foods as drugs. Most of us don't like the taste of medicines and can't think of anything more abhorrent than the idea that our foods are medicines. It's only by realizing that we already do use foods as drugs . . . recreational drugs . . . with all the untoward complications, that we can get our mind around the idea of using foods for their therapeutic effects.

RECREATIONAL EATING

If eating hadn't been enshrined as entertainment before, it is now. Dining out is referred to as the theater of the 1990s. With the explosion in obesity, diet-related cancers, diabetes, and heart disease, it's little wonder that this culinary theater is increasingly a Greek tragedy. The whole idea that we eat for entertainment underscores the idea that foods are recreational drugs. We eat French fries, pancakes dripping with butter and syrup, Big Macs, sugarcoated cereals, and fatty red meats to feel happy, satisfied, energized, celebratory. Unfortunately, we fail to ask this question: If these foods can make us feel good, won't spectacular foods make us feel phenomenal?

Recreational foods can be more dangerous than recreational drugs. If you mainline fried fish and chips, premium ice cream with hot fudge sauce, donuts, and Boston cream pie, you could die a much earlier death than if you smoke marijuana or even if you shoot heroin. Sure, an accidental overdose of heroin could kill you, but obesity and high-fat diets are known risk factors for and accelerators of heart disease and cancer. Food is America's worst drug addiction. Why? Cocaine kills 1,500 a year, heroin another 1,500 and those are the biggest of the big-league drugs. But foods contribute to 70 percent of all deaths in America, killing hundreds of thousands a year.

What's the difference between a diner downing a 16-ounce fat-drenched steak with onion rings at a major steak house and taking a slug of heroin? Dosage. Both are hitting brain cells with opiates. That's right. The big reinforcement for eating high-fat, high-sugar recreational foods is that they set off the release of natural opiates and other pleasure chemicals in the brain . . . strongly reinforcing the use of really awful foods, shows the research of Cornell University's Elliot Blass.

The chronic use of food as recreational drugs sets up distinct patterns in the production of brain chemicals that regulate appetite and mood. You may act a certain way — depressed, low, anxiety stricken — not because it's your personality, but because of the foods you eat. This pattern is self-reinforcing because you must eat terrible foods with great regularity to assuage your food-induced anxiety and depression, only to find that their aftereffects are to reintroduce these same symptoms.

Take as an example the American obsession with quick energy. The usual solution is a caffeine-blasted carbo high, such as a coffee and bagel or cola and pizza. We certainly feel energized, so much so that millions of us do this dozens of times a week. But each evening we feel increasingly hungry, weary, worn down. We are creating our own chronic fatigue–like syndrome. For those of you who don't want to give up the high, let me convince you that you can trade this short-lived burst of energy for a deep, inner, commanding power. Look at the contrast between a caffeine or sugar buzz and the strong therapeutic power of foods. The different energies you'll get from them are represented by Kramer, the character on *Seinfeld,* and Clint Eastwood. Kramer may think he has all the energy in the world but he appears nervous, jittery, hyper, as if he's about to jump out of his skin. Now take Clint Eastwood. In a low deep voice, he says exactly what he means. You can sense he is a deep powerhouse of energy. Imagine how you want to appear in front of your family or coworkers . . . a scatterbrained Kramer, or a collected Clint Eastwood. I used to try and get myself "up" for a broadcast or a speech. I'd take two or three Diet Cokes and be appalled when I looked at myself on the screen . . . not the kind of reassuring, commanding presence I'd want.

Obesity has come to the fore as America's number-one public health emergency. The medical establishment is now recognizing what pioneers like Nathan Pritikin and Dean Ornish did years ago. Our diet is killing us. We are eating a diet to which humans have never adapted and may not adapt for millions of years. In response, our genetic machinery is churning out a record amount of obesity, diabetes, heart disease, and cancer.

If your goal is a vanity-driven improvement in your appearance . . . GREAT! Most of us fall into the trap of feeling it is far better to look good than be good; however, looks are a far stronger motivating factor than ameliorating the risk of disease down the road. With perfect weight control, you'll be struck by an immediate, striking improvement in your health that is effected more powerfully than if you had taken a lifesaving medicine. Remarkable new evidence, accumulated just during the last year, shows that a focus on the here and now, changing foods to feel and look better, has profound consequences for the future. Our waistlines are a daily reminder of our overall health. They are an excellent yardstick of just how well we are doing.

Few of us who haven't encountered grave illness close up really feel the threat seriously enough to make big changes. But aim those changes at our midsection, and our midsection soars. The other motivation will come once you see how great you feel. Your improved temperament, daily attitude, and youthful feel will make it stick on a daily basis.

Terry Shintani, M.D., J.D., M.P.H., a great friend and pioneer of the Eat More to Weigh Less concept, fought a hard battle to save the lives of native Hawaiians. He found weight loss almost incidental to eating a healthier diet. He encourages his patients to look at being overweight as an early sign of bad health and a killer diet. Unfortunately, weight loss in most programs is antithetical to good health.

The following chapters will describe what foods can do to make you thin, by making your brain feel great, turning off hunger, and dropping glucose load. They contain every really great tool you need to control your weight.

part one *The Strategy*

Make Your Brain Feel Great

Think of your brain as a cranky diner. If you wait on it like a diligent maître d', serving every course on time, in precisely the right manner, at the perfect temperature, your brain's hard pressed to become too demanding. But boy, let one course come late or cold and this genius is all over you like a bad suit. When it comes to food and brain chemistry, for every mistaken action there is a damaging, even overwhelming, opposite reaction. Let that brain get low on key hormones, nutrients, and neurochemicals, and it will pounce back with a vengeance, demanding that you pay up quickly with hefty penalties. Feed your brain badly and there's a huge price to be levied in excess calories, poor food choices, lackluster mental performance, and a foul mood. Unfortunately, most of us treat our brains worse than the rudest waiter treats a customer.

Conventional Wisdom
You have to choose between looking good or feeling good.

LEAN
You've got to feel good to look good.

ROAD MAP
Each and every one of us medicates ourselves from dawn to nightcap with cigarettes, diet colas, coffee, over-the-counter drugs, prescription painkillers, candy bars, French fries, hamburgers, pasta, hollandaise sauce . . . you name it, we've done it (well, maybe not all of it). We understand that the only way to have a successful day is for our brains to feel great. This chapter is designed to give you every last

reasonable, legal, safe, and healthy method to make your brain feel great from the moment you wake up until you're fast asleep. You should be able to achieve a terrific mood all day long by eating the right foods so that you have the willpower to lose weight and stay thin. The key is building high enough levels of serotonin, the master weight-control neurotransmitter, in the brain. Add to that the neurotransmitter dopamine to energize yourself and you have a complementary package to adjust and control your mood as you choose.

BUILDING SELF-CONTROL THROUGH THE FOODS YOU EAT

Those who perfectly control their weight display to the world great self-control. However, ask yourself this question: Do you think that you'll gain that degree of self-control by cranking your metabolism down to a low whisper, bringing on pit of the stomach hunger, light-headedness, and blurry vision, while robbing your body of essential nutrients? That's how feared dictators get prisoners to talk. They starve them. How does dieting make your brain feel? Vague and forgetful for starters. Researchers concluded that dieting had approximately the same effect as a couple of drinks, wrecking reaction time and mental calculations. Even worse, Dianne Budd, M.D., of the University of California at San Francisco, found that if normal-sized people limit calories, depression increases, and there's a decrement in critical thinking skills. Says Dr. Budd, "The cognitive performance of people was statistically significantly less while dieting. Also, in a controlled study, the evidence shows that measurable parameters of depression increase such as sleep disorders and loss of libido. Basically, you're dumber when you diet."

If you want willpower, the tried-and-failed behavioral approach will have you thinking noble thoughts to ward off temptation while you starve.

Conventional Wisdom
Good food satisfies the stomach.

LEAN
Great food satisfies the brain.

MOOD CHEMISTRY

The most basic secret to achieving great success in perfect weight control is to make your brain feel great through mood chemistry. Here's how it works. When you eat certain foods, your digestive system breaks them down into individual amino acids. Once these amino acids are absorbed into your bloodstream, specific ones cross into the brain to speed the manufacture of mood-enhancing neurotransmitters, so you are actually changing the chemistry of the part of your brain that controls mood through the foods you eat. Learning how to use the right foods will help you master your self-control while eating and your motivation to exercise. In the process of learning to control your weight, you will achieve an even greater benefit. You will learn how to give your brain a terrific day every day, all day long.

Sarah Leibowitz, Ph.D., professor of behavioral neurobiology at The Rockefeller University and the world's premier authority on the neurobiology of obesity, says, "The brain is where the action is." She has demonstrated that the foods we eat create profound changes in the brain. A high-fat or high-carbohydrate diet changes the actual composition of the brain. There are lower amounts of the neurotransmitters that control positive mood and greater amounts of the hormones that make us overeat, making the brain of an obese person fundamentally different from that of a thin person. These changes are so profound in laboratory animals, they are observed with the very first high-fat meal. The brain of an obese person craves carbos and fats to feed a brain reward system. With each bite of fat, with each extra pound, our control over the brain hormones that make us fat is stolen from us.

I. SEROTONIN: THE MASTER WEIGHT-CONTROL DRUG

Serotonin has become the darling of mood neurotransmitters. Duke University's Redford Williams, M.D., author of *Anger Kills,* says, "Almost everything gets better with increased levels of serotonin." Michael Norden, M.D., author of *Beyond Prozac* and a practicing psychiatrist in Seattle, Washington, asserts that serotonin acts as the brain's police, saying no to drugs, alcohol, binge eating, and impulsive, even criminal behaviors. A serotonin-stripped brain has no chance of resisting the temptations of food to exert any semblance of weight control. Richard Wurtman, M.D., director of the Clinical Research Center at the Massachusetts Institute of Technology, also calls serotonin the master weight-control drug.

More to the point, high serotonin stores are the buffer you want to build against body fat. The more serotonin your brain makes, the fewer excess calories you'll consume and the more likely you'll choose the great foods that will keep you lean. Here's why: Your brain makes a substance called MCH, which causes a ravenous craving for carbohydrates. Even though MCH is made deep in the part of the brain called the hypothalamus, it is released in the frontal lobe, which is where eating decisions are made. The major neurotransmitter for the frontal lobe is serotonin. So when MCH is released, a serotonin-starved brain has little chance of resisting the urge to binge, while a serotonin-rich brain can more easily say no!

Dr. Redford Williams says, "Low levels of serotonin are more than depressing, they're downright dangerous. If you look at the profile of biological behavioral characteristics that hostile and depressed people have, every one of them [is] potentially the result of low brain function." The likely reason these behaviors, such as overeating, high alcohol consumption, and smoking, cluster in hostile and depressed people is that they have low serotonin levels. Dr. Williams suggests that increased anger and irritation, smoking, overeating, obesity, and alcoholism are the result of a single underlying neurochemical condition that he has termed deficit central nervous system serotonin function.

Where's the proof of his hypothesis? Dr. Williams says that there is a considerable body of evidence linking aggressive behaviors with decreased brain serotonin. For example, increasing serotonin in both monkeys and humans decreases hostile and depressive behaviors. Monkeys groom other monkeys more. Monkeys even exhibit human behavior, acting more social or "affiliative" and less isolated with higher levels of serotonin. For violent offenders with antisocial, borderline personality disorder, Prozac raises serotonin levels to decrease their anger. There is also very extensive and convincing evidence that weak brain serotonin function contributes to increased alcohol consumption.

On the flip side, do you wonder how the concepts of too rich and too thin ever became linked? Many of the very rich are indeed very thin for good reason. New social studies show that as you become more successful, your brain makes more serotonin. When Michael McGuire, M.D., director of the nonhuman primate laboratory at UCLA, examined a dominant male monkey before he climbed the social hierarchy, the monkey's serotonin level was unexceptional. But by winning key battles, his social standing increased and his serotonin rose during his ascent. Likewise, when a dominant male suffered a loss of status, his serotonin level dropped. Use this book to build serotonin levels, and you'll gain a sense of magnanimity and wealth beyond many well-known billionaires. You can engineer a great brain day without being wealthier than a rural peasant.

It's no accident that Prozac, an antidepressant that makes more serotonin available to the brain, became the nation's most popular mood drug. Dr. Norden credits our superstressed lifestyle, lack of sleep, natural-light-deprived work spaces, high temperatures, and polluted modern environment with depleting our serotonin levels and theorizes that we live in a world for which we were not designed. Add to that the last decade of relentless corporate cost cutting, overwork, layoffs, and resultant family breakups, and it's little wonder our brain's supply of serotonin is gutted and we've packed on the pounds in a failed attempt to replace it. Without appropriate levels of serotonin we can become irritable, impotent, impulsive, even suicidal . . . and, as a result, overeat. Serotonin also acts as a "stress immunizer" with which we can endure high levels of stress. If you think of a bad day as sailing through choppy seas in a small dinghy, then think of the high serotonin state as plowing through the same seas in a giant ocean liner.

The first step to creating pleasant sensations in the brain is building a bigger store of serotonin through an entire arsenal that ranges from foods and drugs to light boxes and dawn simulators to protect yourself from bingeing on the wrong foods. For most people, the combination of the right foods and devices will be enough. But there are those with abnormally low stores of neurochemicals for whom prescription drugs are a reasonable choice. Since these drugs aim at precisely the same objective, building higher levels of serotonin, you should consider them, with your doctor, if you are dangerously overweight. Danger strikes when you're only 20 percent overweight, putting you at increased risk of diabetes, high blood pressure, or heart disease.

HOW TO BOOST SEROTONIN
TRYPTOPHAN

Tryptophan, a mood-enhancing amino acid present in many foods, is the key building block of serotonin. The more tryptophan in your blood, the more crosses into your brain to make serotonin. Responses to tryptophan vary. Women are more likely to feel calm while men may feel drowsy. Large amounts make both men and women sleepy. Since you can't buy tryptophan over the counter any longer after thirty-eight people died of an adverse reaction to a contaminated batch of the product, carbohydrates have become the chief way of mainlining the stuff because they speed the brain's uptake of tryptophan.

CARBOHYDRATES

While Prozac can take weeks to build up stores of serotonin, a high-carbo meal builds up big stores in a matter of minutes. The more carbohydrate you eat, the more tryptophan there is in the blood, the more serotonin your brain makes. Here's an example of using carbohydrate as a drug: A recent Harvard/MIT study used carbohydrates to treat the dysphoria associated with the premenstrual syndrome. The 245 participants met rigorous diagnostic criteria for PMS. Women who drank an experimental mixture containing the carbohydrates dextrose and maltodextrin experienced a significant decrease in anger, depression, confusion, and carbohydrate craving 90 to 180 minutes after ingestion. Although the results were less dramatic than drug therapy, there were also fewer side effects. This drink, PMS Escape, is manufactured by InterNutria of Lexington, Massachusetts.

If you are substantially overweight you may notice little effect of

small amounts of carbohydrate on your mood. MIT's Judith Wurtman, Ph.D., has shown overfat people don't transport tryptophan efficiently into the brain. As a result, an overfat person must eat
enormous amounts of carbohydrates to build much serotonin. For
this reason, if you are substantially overweight, you may need to rely
on other measures to improve serotonin stores, including drugs.
However, with each pound you lose, you will become more sensitive
to the druglike effects of foods, so you can eat less of them to feel
great.

What Kind of Carbohydrate

Be sure to eat carbohydrates that are absorbed slowly into your bloodstream. That assures you of a long-lasting effect. In this way, the tryptophan is stripped out by your digestive processes and sent on its way
into your brain in a slow continuous fashion that avoids caloric excess. Examples are corn tortillas with beans, high-fiber cereals, dense
whole grain breads, and high-quality oatmeal. More of these foods
are listed in the chapters "Hard Grains" and "Hard Fibers."

Carbos to Avoid

Refined carbohydrates such as those in white flour breads, bagels,
muffins, and snack foods are digested quickly and cause a large rise in
blood sugar. While you'll notice the fastest impact on seratonin levels, this is a short-lived strategy and can cause rapid gains in weight.
These foods are the dietary equivalent of "crack," since you'd
have to hammer yourself all day long with them to keep feeling good.
Dr. Michael Norden says the idea "that we should let people have
their cake and muffins just hasn't worked. I've tried it on people and
they simply end up feeling worse — sluggish and gaining weight." By
waiting for the appearance of a symptom, like anxiety or fatigue, you
invent a special need that you are now pressed to extinguish with
megadoses of quick-acting cracklike carbos. The muffin, cake, or
bagel will get you a temporary increase in serotonin, which is immediately calming. But just like having an occasional drink, which will
reduce your stress, having it too often will run your system down. Dr.
Norden explains that the boost in serotonin from a muffin is like the

boost we get from sugar. We quickly get a response and then we crash. There's very little difference in terms of how your body responds to French bread, cornflakes, cakes, bagels, muffins, or table sugar. Most of the refined carbohydrates will give you a surge in blood sugar level, then a huge insulin release followed by the crash. By eating slowly digested carbos such as home-cooked oatmeal, on an empty stomach, you'll continually make serotonin over the course of many hours. That will give you a much more mellow and still powerful feeling than the short-lived rush of the Twinkie high. If you badly need a serotonin fix and do wolf down refined carbos, just eat a single serving. Follow that up with slowly digested carbo so that your blood sugar doesn't dive and you don't create more craving during the rest of the day. For instance, if you have a soft drink, follow it with a bean and whole grain chaser.

NATURAL SEROTONIN BOOSTERS

Light and darkness dominate the rhythm of life on earth. Your health, mood, and behavior all improve with the quality and quantity of sunlight you receive, as does your ability to fall asleep and stay asleep. Yet again, our ancestors had it right: Rising every day at dawn to work or play outdoors in the natural light is what our bodies were designed for. Early to bed, early to rise may not make you rich, but it will give you the great wealth of feeling terrific. Contrast that life of light to the way we live today. The Center of Environmental Therapeutics educates the public about environmental interventions for fatigue, depression, and stress. They say, "We race to work, day or night, summer or winter, comfortably seated inside a convenient mode of transport with tinted windows or curtains, to meet our inflexible appointments and complete our rigid schedules within artificially lighted and artificially ventilated workplaces. Our modern cubicles, deficient in sunlight and fresh air, result in daytime fatigue and reduced work performance, increased accident rates and sick days, dietary imbalance and weight gain, insomnia and depression."

Boy, that's a mouthful, but how true. I think of our offices on West 57th Street, which are windowless, fed with recycled air, and sprayed with the electromagnetic radiation of a major broadcasting facility. I swear the building seems to make people depressed and physically ill. I wondered why we all feel so much better on the road, even if it's in Bosnia. The answer is light and fresh air. With our natural rhythms thrown out of whack, it's no wonder you see most of us piling those extra junk carbos onto our cafeteria trays. By overeating, we're desperately trying to make up for the serotonin that's been robbed from our systems by the environment. Increase brain serotonin levels and you decrease your craving for carbohydrates. The higher you can push your brain serotonin without resorting to foods, the less food you have to eat.

There are two completely natural ways of restoring the serotonin that our modern work environment robs from our system: light therapy and negative ion generators. The more serotonin you can build with these therapies, the less carbohydrate you have to eat to get the same effect. If you gain five to ten pounds every winter, this is the ticket to preserving your waistline all winter long.

LIGHT THERAPY

Artificial lights have been a major treatment of winter depression for ten years. The biggest recent innovation is a substantial increase in the intensity of light therapy, which reduces the duration of treatment sessions to 30 minutes a day of bright light. Columbia University's Michael Terman, Ph.D., says, "Within several days of exposure to bright light treatment, these vegetative symptoms along with the dysphoric mood can vanish entirely. This contrasts with standard medication treatment for depression which can take weeks for blood levels to establish confidently a therapeutic effect. This is a very quick action and makes us think that we're getting to the heart of the mechanism of action. There is a true light deprivation syndrome." If light deprivation in your workplace is creating feelings of lethargy or outright depression, you may want to consider light therapy with your physician.

How does this relate to serotonin? The theory is that exposure to light stimulates serotonin availability in the nervous system in much the same way the serotonin re-uptake inhibitors like Prozac do. Dr. Terman says, "This is an indication that the light is working on the serotonin system. There's definitely a normalization of the serotonin response as people are relieved of their depressive symptoms." The most striking evidence of light therapy's effect on serotonin was a study in the *Archives of General Psychiatry* of patients who had gotten better with light treatment. Researchers then rapidly depleted their brain tryptophan down to 20 percent of normal levels, presumably reducing their brain serotonin levels. The patients became depressed again. "This serves as further evidence that light is working directly on serotonin," says Raymond Lam, M.D., director of the Mood Disorders Clinic at the Vancouver Hospital and Health Sciences Center. (And with Vancouver's weather, he should know!)

This is the most convincing evidence that light therapy can boost your serotonin levels to cut your craving for carbohydrates and give you control over what you eat. There are three major light dosing factors: level, duration, and time of day. You will need to experiment to discover what works best for you. The most state-of-the-art light therapy produces a 10,000 lux level, which can work in sessions as short as thirty minutes and cost as little as $425. Lower levels of lux require longer exposure, but cost less money. Morning is a highly effective time to use light therapy, but your doctor can discuss the proper time of day for you.

Dawn Simulation Therapy

Dawn simulation, the next generation of light therapy, is the slow, gradual transition from dark to light. Like "real" dawn, this subtle light gradually penetrates the eyelids to wake you up. Dr. Michael Terman, who introduced dawn simulation, says, "We designed a sophisticated computer system that knows exactly how much light to expect outside at any latitude on earth, at any day of the year and at any time of the day. By using such an artificial light source system, which is much lower in intensity than that used for bright light therapy, in the bedroom, we can create a dawn signal that would mimic, for example, a gradual sunrise in May, in the middle of February. We have exposed people to this system for a matter of days and found that they begin to wake up spontaneously, automatically, earlier than before and uniformly showing greater morning alertness and energy with an antidepressant effect within one week's time, which is comparable with bright light treatment."

With such strong evidence for the use of light therapy, you could consider it if you experience large winter weight gain, especially if linked to depressive symptoms. If you live in an industrial cave, as I do, which is light deprived year round, you could consider using therapeutic lights at work. I set up a full-strength light box at my desk during the winter to maintain my serotonin stores and my sanity. Make certain to use a well-designed light box, like those mentioned in the appendix, and not an inexpensive gimmick out of a trendy catalog.

The Center for Environmental Therapeutics also offers these suggestions to get more light:

- Get outside as much as possible.
- Adapt your interior spaces to maximize lighting. Clear the windows with exposures toward the sun. Keep light fixtures not more than three feet away from your work and relaxation areas. Substitute the newer fluorescent lamps of similar wattage to increase the amount of light without increasing your energy bills.
- Minimize the use of sunglasses except when you absolutely need them.

NEGATIVE ION THERAPY

All right, I'll admit it. Negative ion therapy does sound more than a little bit looney, but hear me out. Do you know the sense of well-being you have after a thunderstorm or in the fresh air near the ocean or a waterfall? What you're getting is a healthy dose of negative ions. Those ions make neurons in the brain more responsive to serotonin. So, as an example, a thunderstorm improves your mood almost like an electronic pulse of Prozac. Contrast that to the poor mental state and sickness that sweeps through Europe with the hot winds from the Sahara called the foehn or the Santa Ana winds in Southern California, which leave you awash with positive ions and the attendant ill effects. Positive ions make neurons in the brain less responsive to serotonin, so you may feel down when these hot winds blow through. Unfortunately, the United States and other industrialized nations replicate the black mood of the foehn and the Santa Ana by heavily polluting the air with positive ions from computers and electromagnetic waves from electrical devices or sucking out negative ions with air-recycling machines. In fact, the most ubiquitous source of gloom-inducing positive ions are cathode ray computer screens. Enter the negative ion machine. Dr. Michael Terman of Columbia University found that negative ion therapy relieved depression and irritability while improving cognitive performance and energy by decreasing the number of positive ions. I keep one next to my computer. You only need to be exposed to the light for a short amount of time. "Most people think you only receive the benefits for only as long as you're exposed to the light or ion generator. But, all of these methods have a pervasive 24-hour effect on physiology. Although the push may take place in the morning, the change is measurable throughout the day," says Dr. Terman.

The appendix lists negative ion machines recommended by Dr. Terman.

STRESS REDUCTION

While hunger is a strong impetus to replenish serotonin, stress is equally strong. Stress robs the brain of serotonin. The more you decrease your stress, the lower your need for foods to rebuild serotonin stores. The best stress reduction is attained through regular aerobic exercise, as determined by a large battery of tests at the Massachusetts General Hospital. Dr. Dean Ornish uses meditation as a stress reducer in his weight loss and reversing heart disease programs. A big part of his success in weight loss, I believe, is keeping stress levels low enough to reduce the excessive need for food-based serotonin fortification in the form of junk food and refined sugars. Zen followers have published research showing that their form of meditation improves serotonin stores as well.

SLEEP

There is no way to control your weight without the proper amount and quality of sleep. Dr. Woodrow Weiss, codirector of the sleep disorders center at Beth Israel Deaconess Medical Center and an associate professor at Harvard Medical School, demonstrated sleepiness was tightly linked to weight gains in a study of 508 men. A brain gnawing at you for more sleep will allow you only one easy out: more food . . . lots more. Now this may seem like a simple point, but you must eat the right foods to set up a good night's sleep. By tweaking your physiology, you can prepare your body for sleep. You may not be aware of the effect of food, but try this experiment so you do become more aware. Eat a big protein meal, preferably steak, about an hour before your bedtime. Count how many times during the night you find yourself slightly awake. Also count how many times you have to pee. Judge how groggy or awake you feel the next morning. Also note your pulse when you are about to fall asleep and then when you wake during the night. My experience is that my pulse is a good 15 beats higher, that I wake five or more times during the night. Now prepare for the next evening by eating a big lunch, a moderate midafternoon snack, and then a light evening snack instead of dinner. See if you don't have a far sounder night's sleep. You're really accomplishing two objectives. The first is to allow your body to lose weight during the night by feeding off body fat stores instead of food left in your stomach. The second is to wake up refreshed enough to make the tough food choices. Remember, too, that your body is restoring your serotonin stores during sleep.

DRUGS

Conventional antidepressants that boost serotonin levels can have a mild effect on weight loss, by decreasing the length of a meal. When Prozac was tested as a weight-loss drug, high doses had to be given to achieve weight loss, creating significant side effects. Michael Devlin, M.D., a research psychiatrist at the New York State Psychiatric Institute, says, "Prozac was found to decrease eating time — you got fuller faster. There was a real dose-response relationship. Daily doses of 60–80 mg. were more effective than daily doses of 20 mg." Prozac only continues to work effectively to aid weight loss if it is part of a nutrition and exercise program.

The newly approved drug Dexfenfluramine increases serotonin for serious weight loss in three separate ways: First, it spurs the release of serotonin; second, it prevents the re-uptake of serotonin so that more remains around the nerve endings longer; third, it directly stimulates the serotonin receptor. Since serotonin is the predominant neurotransmitter in the frontal lobe where the decision to eat is made, you would expect to gain greater control over food intake with serotonin.

Studies conducted by Richard Wurtman, M.D., showed that Dexfenfluramine specifically reduced the graving for carbohydrates. The drug also has potent effects on mood, acting as an antidepressant, but requiring far smaller doses than Prozac. The drug appears to alleviate the desire to consume large quantities of food. People taking Dexfenfluramine have experienced "getting full" faster. However, a *New England Journal of Medicine* report found that one in 20,000 users suffers primary pulmonary hypertension, an often fatal condition. More studies are needed to confirm just how great this danger really is. That makes Dexfenfluramine a drug to be considered only by those who are at least 20 percent overweight and suffer diabetes, hypertension, or heart disease. Now under FDA scrutiny is another serotonin-enhancing drug called Meridia (sibutramine hydrochloride monohydrate). Manufactured by Knoll Pharmaceuticals, Meridia increases brain serotonin and norepinephrine, the two chemicals involved in appetite control. In clinical trials the drug has been shown to reduce patients' weight by at least 5 to 10 percent. Most recently, however, an FDA advisory committee voted 5 to 4 against approval of the drug because of an increase in hypertension in people who took it. FDA spokeswoman Susan Cruzan says, "Now, the company needs to go back and conduct other studies to determine if there's a subgroup of people for whom the drug is absolutely safe."

CUT DOWN ON ASPARTAME

Among the postdrug, postalcohol, postnicotine baby boomers, the caffeine/aspartame (NutraSweet) combination is the last really great drug high. I'll be the first to admit that I love a Diet Coke. The caffeine/aspartame formulation feels like rocket fuel for the brain for clean-living people, with far stronger effects than either ingredient alone. The caffeine acts as a stimulant, while aspartame directly affects the brain's internal reward pathways. It works even better when you're already feeling great. But watch out! There are now reports of mild depression following the use of aspartame. By late afternoon you may find the aspartame's by-products leave you mildly anxious and even depressed. The Aspartame Consumer Safety Network, a nonprofit consumer advocacy group against the use of aspartame, concludes that aspartame causes a blockage in the formation of serotonin in the brain. The group's fact sheet states, "Many people who don't make enough serotonin from their food are more susceptible to insomnia, depression, and/or PMS. If these genetically deficient people are also swallowing aspartame, they will more readily have headaches, insomnia, depression, hostility, anxiety, and a host of other negative symptoms." Aspartame and caffeine feed into an addictive nature.

The more important question is: Will aspartame help you lose weight? Dr. Robin Kanarek of Tufts says, "Products containing artificial sweeteners may prompt people to eat more than if they never even consumed a sweetened product to begin with." Compared to water, drinks containing aspartame increased feelings of hunger and the desire to eat and reduced feelings of fullness. Similar effects were seen with saccharin and Acesulfame K. Michael Jacobson, Ph.D., of the Center for Science in the Public Interest, says, "Obesity has skyrocketed along with the use of aspartame." It's certainly not a magic bullet. "There's little evidence that drinking an aspartame-containing beverage in any way helps you lose weight," he says.

BOOST YOUR PROSTAGLANDINS

Prostaglandins are master hormones produced in all cells. Prostaglandin production is heavily dependent on what you eat. And depending on what you eat your body can produce good prostaglandins, which appear to increase the effects of brain serotonin, dampen pain, and promote immune response, or bad ones, which are associated with high levels of insulin, carbohydrate cravings, depression, and weight gain. Dr. Norden says, "Some of the most remarkable improvements in depression I have seen in my practice have come from enhancing the amount of good prostaglandins through diet." Laboratory evidence that bad prostaglandins are elevated in people who have depression has been remarkably consistent.

The science of making good prostaglandins to boost your serotonin is a young one, and the measures you could take to make them could become a full-time hobby. There are, however, a few simple measures that will boost your good prostaglandin production. These are all measures I'd recommend even if you don't buy the still controversial prostaglandin hypothesis.

FISH OIL   The oil in cold saltwater fish like salmon, mackerel, herring, tuna, and sardines increases the good prostaglandins. The healthful oil is best eaten in fish and not in capsules. Experts believe that Omega 3 fatty acids are potent promoters of making the brain feel great. This may be why they're called brain food.

AVOID TRANSFATTY ACIDS   These increase the number of bad prostaglandins. Many baked goods and all foods labeled as using hydrogenated or partially hydrogenated fats contain transfatty acids.

AVOID BEEF FAT AND EGG YOLKS   Both contain high levels of arachidonic acid, which is the key precursor for bad prostaglandins and for a recently discovered hormone that makes new fat cells. Some speculate that the reason fatty red meats and egg yolks are bad for you has less to do with their fatty acid content and more to do with the boost they give to bad prostaglandin production. Since the arachidonic acid is in beef fat, you can eat lean red meat if you trim the fat and eat lean grades.

PROTEIN   Eat some protein with every meal and snack. This releases more of the hormone glucagon, which counters the effects of insulin. Check your protein intake to be certain you are getting enough.

AVOID CAFFEINE

LOW INSULIN   Keep your insulin level low and steady by following the measures in the chapter "Drop Your Glucose Load." Low insulin levels promote good prostaglandin production, while high insulin levels are the strongest possible promoter of bad prostaglandins. This measure alone is the most important one you can make.

In summary, the more serotonin you can build through slowly digested carbos, light boxes, therapeutic drugs, negative ion generators, relaxation and a good night's sleep, the less you'll have to overeat to achieve the same effect.

2. DOPAMINE: THE MASTER ENERGIZER

The neurotransmitter dopamine creates mental energy, vigilance, and alertness. As your brain's dopamine neurons light up, you can feel yourself becoming more positive, growing more buoyant, even cheerful. This is the neurotransmitter you'll want to get going in the morning, to be more aggressive at work (in a nice way!), or to work harder longer without fatigue. Dopamine will give you the motivation to exercise longer. One longtime broadcast associate of mine lost fifteen pounds in five weeks by turning her dopamine on. It gave her the energy to walk to and from work and bike regularly on the weekends.

HOW TO BOOST DOPAMINE

The amino acid tyrosine is the key building block of dopamine. When subjects received tyrosine, complex cognitive performances such as learning and memory appeared to improve as did reaction time and vigilance. Fatigue and depression also were relieved. The subsequent rise in brain dopamine leads to increased vigor and energy and increases your concentration. There's little wonder that the National Academy of Sciences has studied tyrosine for use in combat rations for the United States Armed Forces. Experts believe that when you are under severe stress, your brain's neurons are fired more frequently. The availability of extra tyrosine appears to increase dopamine release and improve behavior. In humans, tyrosine has been shown to reduce adverse behavioral effects associated with stress. Supplemental doses of 85 to 170 mg restored performance and mood and relieved symptoms among those exposed to physical stresses. Tyrosine supplements are available without a prescription in health food stores; however, I recommend a protein-rich meal as the most practical, satisfactory, and natural means of increasing brain levels of tyrosine.

Foods High in Tyrosine

Food	Amount	Tyrosine (milligrams)
Soybeans	1 cup	2,000
1% cottage cheese	1 cup	1,492
Skim mozzarella	2 oz.	794
Chicken	2 oz.	590
Fish	2 oz.	490
Beef	2 oz.	470
Egg	1	250

Cheeses are also densely packed with tyrosine, which is why it's so hard to fall asleep at night after eating cheeses. You can see that just two ounces of skim mozzarella provides more tyrosine (794 mg) than two ounces of beef, chicken, or fish.

While there is a several-fold increase in serotonin levels after a carbohydrate meal, dopamine is more difficult to make. There is only a 60 percent increase in dopamine after a protein meal, so the most potent means of producing more tyrosine in your brain to boost dopamine levels is to eat your cheese, soybeans, chicken, fish, or beef on an empty stomach without any accompanying carbohydrates, advises MIT's Dr. Richard Wurtman.

BALANCE

Think of tryptophan and tyrosine at opposite ends of a seesaw. Tryptophan is calming while tyrosine is alerting. The more carbos in a meal, the more tryptophan predominates, the more relaxed, calm, or (in large doses) sleepy you'll be. The more protein in a meal, the more tyrosine predominates, the more alert you'll become. The heart of changing your mood during any given day is varying the amounts of carbohydrate and protein to make yourself more alert or calm. Protein-rich foods from breakfast through early afternoon are the best way to make your workday productive. Be warned, however, that just eating protein for an entire day will block serotonin production to the point that you may crave carbos severely enough to overeat. I follow a big morning protein load like skim milk or a protein shake with a bowl of oatmeal or high-fiber cereal. Because the cereals are slowly digested, the carbos will have a very modest blunting effect on dopamine production and still allow you to make enough serotonin to feel calm and relaxed.

SEX

I asked Richard Kogan, M.D., acting director of the Human Sexuality Program at New York Hospital–Cornell Medical Center the question: How can I produce more dopamine? "Have more sex! Sex is fabulous for us. It's incredibly good. Basically, there's little down side to it. People who have active sex lives have more powerful and better functioning immune systems. They are less prone to a whole host of mental disorders. Sexual health is extremely positive." When male rats have orgasms, a tremendous amount of dopamine is released into the synapse. Male rats that became more sexually active, in experiments performed by Jozsef Knoll, became thinner and lived longer. Perhaps that's how the dieter's slogan "Reach for your mate instead of your plate" came about. Sex is a proven method of making more dopamine.

PHARMACEUTICALS

There is a highly spirited competition among pharmaceutical manufacturers to find drugs that increase dopamine stores. Upjohn is the current leader. Older drugs that boost dopamine are of the amphetamine class and are considered ineffective in the long term and potentially dangerous. Also Dexfenfluramine stimulates serotonin-loaded nerve endings to trigger nerves loaded with dopamine.

3. ENDORPHINS: NATURAL ECSTASY

Our lives are dominated by body rhythms that give our days natural highs and lows. In the wee hours of the morning, our hormones are uniquely timed to gently begin prodding the body toward dawn. Our waking hormones crescendo during the day, reaching a natural peak in midafternoon. Rock stars have long tried to improve upon these natural, delicate rhythms by using drugs from amphetamines to cocaine to build towering peaks to their days, then cushioning the fall into the darkest valleys with comforting downers from Quaaludes to Valium. It's little wonder that the era of junk food is also the era of sex, drugs, and rock 'n' roll. In fact, ethnobotanist Gary Nabhan calls today's junk food diet the culinary equivalent of quick sex. Even those of us with more puritanical and drug-free backgrounds still demand the "I want it now" druglike effects of food on our moods. The primary villain is a blood sugar level that rises and falls throughout the day in wild swings from very high to quite low. The body has its own opiates, called endorphins, which produce a calm, euphoric high. Unfortunately, the easiest way to make more endorphins is by eating refined starches such as white flour breads, cereals, bagels, and pastas, according to Luke Bucci, Ph.D., vice president of research at Weider Nutrition Group in Salt Lake City, Utah. "Sugar is a trigger. Without any fiber, starches are just like sugar to the brain. That's why these people are hooked on these carbohydrate diets. It's an addiction. But it's the bad carbohydrate, not the natural grains and the beans and the whole foods," he says. Curiously, the glucose receptor is closely tied to the endorphin system. For survival, the brain of primitive man needed to be rewarded for the intake of small amounts of sugars imbedded in fruits and vegetables so the body would know to eat them. But basic brain design could in no way have anticipated the advent of the Twinkie. Still, there are natural ways to make your brain feel great by making more endorphins without bingeing on junk foods.

HOW TO BOOST ENDORPHINS

Exercise: I admit it. You thought that as a lifelong aerobic animal I'd sneak this in and I did. Exercise is the primary alternative method of creating the ultimate feel-good brain chemicals, endorphins. Thirty minutes or more of exercise can give you the same endorphin high as a chocolate bar, but it will last all day, not just a matter of minutes. The best way to make your brain feel great for the majority of the day is to do your workout in the morning. This picks you up by the bootstraps and delivers you to a great new day. The "runner's high" endorphins generated by exercise will continue to give you a high over the course of the rest of the day. I like morning exercise because it gives a double "high" to your day. Morning exercise provides a natural early spike so your body's clock will generate hormones to reach your natural high in the afternoon. Since you will continue to burn calories long after you stop exercises, morning is an ideal time to garner the daylong effect of a higher metabolism. It makes you a high-energy person. The chapter "Fat-Ripping Exercises" has a complete list of the best weight-loss exercises.

Foods can help make that happen in a major way by preparing your body for exercise and are described in the chapter "Feedforward Eating." There are also some highly intriguing but still experimental supplements that can boost endorphins and cut the craving for junk food.

Having a great day all day is the true wealth in life and you can do it without a six-figure income. The best meals are peasant dishes that cost only a few dollars a day. Spend a morning in Dhaka, the capital city of Bangladesh. These are among the poorest people on earth. You may be tempted to reassure yourself how much happier you are coming from a life of relative opulence in America. But as you look at happy faces brimming with laughter wherever you look, think that on a plant-based diet, they may feel a great deal better than you've ever felt. When I eat the foods of the Bengals I feel as good as I can remember. You can feel as good as a human being can feel . . . better than you have at any time for years. With each passing day you will feel an accumulating sense of well-being and joy.

This chapter has covered only half of making your brain feel great; the other half is found in the next chapter, which will help you cut your hunger and your cravings for food.

Turn Off Hunger

"These smells are pleasant when we are hungry, but when we are sated and not requiring to eat, they are not pleasant." Sounds like Aristotle made this appraisal at a lumberjacks' all-you-can-eat breakfast. He observed that if foods taste good, we like them and want more, but only to a point . . . like the forty-second flapjack. Several millennia later, research confirms that the pleasantness of taste declines during consumption. But that can take forever if you're eating Lay's potato chips. What Aristotle didn't appreciate is that we have different hungers and tastes that must be sated. As we've all learned the hard way, when the waiter proffers the dessert menu, you may have sated many hungers but not the sweet one. You must satisfy them all.

Hunger is one of nature's strongest forces, so cutting hunger is no idle task. Hunger is driven by the taste, smell, even the appearance of food. A small amount of hunger is dangerous stuff when it comes to controlling the impulse to eat. Hunger should be avoided if you want to become lean. It's a signal you've eaten the wrong foods at the wrong times. Some foods spur you to take on thousands more calories than you ever intended; others can cut consumption by hundreds of calories in a single meal and nearly 1,500 a day.

Conventional Wisdom
An empty stomach makes you thin.

LEAN
A full stomach makes you thin.

ROAD MAP

This chapter has the most effective measures known to help you kill your hunger. Foods can trip different signal systems to cut down your urge to eat. Some work directly by pure mechanical stretching of the stomach. That's covered in the section "Satisfy the Stomach." Others are far more sophisticated, involving complex signals to the brain that cut the craving for specific foods. They're covered in the section "Satisfy the Brain."

If you doubt your ability to eat foods that cut your hunger, just think of how you feel the morning after overstuffing yourself at a Thanksgiving meal. You've got so much food jammed into your intestine that you still feel chock-full fourteen hours later. Now imagine creating the same satiety with far fewer calories.

By choosing foods that quickly cut your hunger, you have a remarkable tool for controlling your weight since you will consume far fewer calories at that meal and the next. Want proof? A classic study involved the comparison of eating whole wheat bread versus white bread. One group was given whole wheat bread, while the other was given white bread and both were told to eat as much as they wanted until they were full. The whole wheat group ate far fewer calories than the white bread group, even though both groups were equally satisfied. Why? The whole wheat bread had far more fiber so it was much more filling and had far less effect on elevating blood sugar so it caused far less hunger.

PROOF OF CONCEPT

The University of Sydney in Australia undertook research to prove that some foods make you satisfied longer than others. Their report in the *European Journal of Clinical Nutrition* used a "satiety index." The researchers asked participants how hungry they were every fifteen minutes for two hours after eating a 240-calorie serving of a food. As an example, oatmeal has been shown to be twice as filling as white bread, three times as filling as a donut, and almost five times as filling as a croissant. Among the most satisfying foods were fish, porridge, apples, oranges, brown pasta, and beans. The least satisfying foods were cookies, white pasta, bananas, cornflakes, French fries, white bread, ice cream, yogurt, peanuts, donuts, cake, and croissants. As a final note, remember that hunger has a purpose beyond making sure you eat enough calories. MIT's Judith Wurtman, Ph.D., says, "Cravings are a way of our brain and body telling us that we should be eating certain foods." The strongest hungers are driven by the need to make more of a specific hormone or neurotransmitter. However, if you give the body exactly what it needs, before it wants it, you kill the cravings and cut the calories.

SATISFY THE STOMACH

The stomach is ground zero when it comes to a targeting priority for the druglike effect of foods on weight control. Certain foods are slow to be released from the stomach into the small intestine; they can slow the absorption of sugars into the bloodstream and stretch the stomach to signal the brain it is full. If you're going for the gold, this is it.

FILL 'ER UP

Twenty years ago stomach-stapling operations gained great popularity because of their ability to limit the volume that the stomach could hold when full. There was even an experimental effort to put a balloon into the stomach to keep it partly full. But there is another more practical solution. Use foods to fill up. Isn't that how you get fat? you might ask? Sure, if they're foods that make you fat. But if you eat foods that are low in calories and imbued with special filling qualities, you hit a win/win situation. That means high-fiber foods. Any high-fiber foods are bulkier, have fewer calories, and take longer to eat, giving your brain a chance to register your food intake before you overeat. For example, you can eat an entire plate of vegetables, but not consume more than 200 calories because high-fiber foods have low-calorie density. Fiber physically separates digestive enzymes from the food they're digesting, which slows down the overall digestive process. A lack of fiber plays a central role in obesity. There's little wonder low-fiber diets give rise to great weight gain. As you follow the decline in fiber consumed from the last century to the present, you will see a corresponding increase in obesity. If you try to control your weight without fiber, you will run a desperate daylong battle against hunger. You will never be truly full and you'll wait uneasily until your next meal arrives. Fiber is the foundation upon which any successful long-term weight control is built. Without it you'll never stand a chance.

1. SOLUBLE FIBER

Fiber is that part of a plant which cannot be digested by the small intestine and is classified as soluble and insoluble. Soluble fibers are so named for their ability to dissolve in water, giving them a big advantage in sopping up liquids. Insoluble fibers are characterized by their inability to dissolve in water. These definitions, however, don't lend any further understanding of their weight-loss properties. It is soluble fiber that is the king of filler-uppers. Here are the demonstrated weight control effects of soluble fiber.

SLOW DOWN STOMACH EMPTYING   No food substance is a more important weapon than the gums found in high-soluble-fiber foods. To convince yourself, try this experiment. You will need a teaspoon of sugar, a stick of chewing gum, and a stopwatch. First put the teaspoon of sugar under your tongue, then time how long the sweet taste stays in your mouth. Now put the stick of gum in your mouth and chew vigorously. With the stopwatch, time how long the sweet taste stays in your mouth. You will find that the gum keeps a sweet taste in your mouth up to ten times longer because the gum acted as a slow-release substance, holding on to the sugar and doling it out more slowly than sugar from the teaspoon.

Soluble fiber in your stomach works just like the chewing gum in your mouth, by delaying stomach emptying and causing food to stay in the stomach longer. That's good for us because a full stomach sends strong satiety signals that shut off further eating. Think of soluble fibers as forming a mucous layer along the lining of your intestine to slow food absorption. Once water and soluble fiber mix in the gut, the stomach and intestine quickly expand. The more fiber you load up on early in a meal and early in the day, the more effectively you kill hunger into the evening hours where it counts the most. Here's a brief sample of high-soluble-fiber foods. The chapter "Hard Fibers" lists them all. The number on the right is the total grams of soluble fiber found in roughly 400 calories. These foods are ranked from the highest amount, 10.5 grams, to the lowest on the list, 4 grams, which is still considered quite a large amount. Beans and high-fiber cereals are the two biggest sources of soluble fiber. In this and other lists it may appear curious that the fiber value for beans is listed as "uncooked." Here's why. Reliable measurements are extraordinarily hard to come by and are made only for the uncooked state. Since the preparation of beans degrades the amount of fiber precipitously, cooked values for beans would be notoriously unreliable. As we'll discuss later, the more beans are mushed or boiled, the lower their soluble-fiber content.

Foods High in Soluble Fiber

Item	Grams of soluble fiber per 400 calorie serving
Heartwise (cereal)	10.5
Benefit (cereal)	10.1
Oat Bran Crunch (cereal)	9.3
Oat bran and oat germ	7.6
Pinto beans, dried, uncooked	7.5
Kidney beans, dark red, dried, uncooked	6.9
Soybeans, dried, uncooked	6.8
Butter beans, dried, uncooked	6.3
Flour, oat	5.5
Oat Bran Cereal (cold)	5.2
All Bran (cereal)	5.1
Oatmeal, uncooked	4.9
Oat Bran Hot Cereal, Apples & Cinnamon, uncooked	4.8
Crispy Oats (cereal)	4.5
Apricots, dried	4.4
White beans, Great Northern, dried, uncooked	4.4
Cheerios (cereal)	4.2
Fruit and Fitness (cereal)	4.2
Common Sense (cereal)	4.1
Figs, dried	4

This table is reprinted with permission from the HCF Nutrition Research Foundation, Inc.

LOWER BLOOD SUGAR LEVELS   Foods rich in soluble fibers lower the absorption of sugar from the small intestine into the bloodstream, creating a smaller appetite and avoiding the nasty low blood sugar which precipitates ravenous hunger.

DUMP EXTRA CALORIES   Gums cause maldigestion and malabsorption of carbohydrates. Some are dumped into the stool and passed out of the body, meaning you got to enjoy eating them without adding inches to your waistline. Fiber also acts to decrease fat absorption.

SUPPRESS APPETITE   When soluble fibers and unspent carbohydrates reach the large colon, they are fermented. The end product is a short-chain fatty acid. Although many long-chain fatty acids are potent fomenters of heart disease, short-chain fatty acids act as a likely appetite suppressant, according to Al Levine of the University of Minnesota. Research also suggests a role for short-chain fatty acids in colon cancer prevention and lowering of blood fats.

CONTROL   The aspect of soluble fibers that I have become most impressed with is the spectacular control they give you over impulse eating. Since you feel so full, you really can say no. I have a big burst of soluble fibers in the early afternoon so I don't overeat at dinner or in the evening. I have found it the single most valuable tool for weight control. It's one thing to will yourself to eat less; it's another to feel full enough to say no.

If you currently have a low-fiber diet, start eating high-soluble-fiber foods slowly. A cup of beans rich in soluble fiber can make you uncomfortably full for many hours. Gums are so powerful that you may still feel full twelve hours later. You may even feel guilty that you've eaten too much. What will surprise you is that you are far fuller on just 300 calories of beans than you ever would be on 1,500 calories of prime rib and potatoes. The soluble fibers are pulling water into them, creating even more bulk and a greater sense of fullness in the upper intestine. To avoid this sense of discomfort, begin by eating no more than a half of a cup per day. Increase your ration of beans by one quarter cup every several days until you reach one and a half cups. If you have eaten lots of high-fiber foods and failed to get the effect that you've just read about, take a close look at the kind of fiber you've been eating. Most processed foods are notoriously poor in soluble fiber and have been processed to the point where they just don't work. See the complete list of high-soluble-fiber foods in the chapter "Hard Fibers." Soluble fiber is maximally effective when taken 10-20 minutes before a meal. You just won't be as hungry, so you won't be able to eat as much when you sit down at the table.

2. HIGH-BULK FOODS

High-bulk foods weigh a great deal but contain very few calories, so they fill you because of their enormous volume. For instance, one pound of cucumbers contains only 76 calories. Four pounds of cucumbers would leave you feeling ready to explode, yet you would have eaten only 324 calories. Where a small amount of a high-fiber food would fill you up, huge quantities of high-bulk foods are necessary.

Terry Shintani, M.D., J.D., M.P.H., pioneered the idea of high-bulk foods for weight loss. He took me through his Wai'anae Coast Comprehensive Health Center where he deals with an overwhelming obesity problem in native Hawaiians. He had a very simple solution. Fill 'er up with high-bulk foods. Terry even developed an "Eat More Index" (EMI), to highlight bulky foods. It is published in full in his book, *Dr. Shintani's Eat More Weigh Less™ Diet*. The higher the number, the fewer the calories per pound. Here is a list of the highest-bulk foods, which are characterized by the fewest calories per pound. The "EMI" figure discloses the numbers of pounds of the food you must eat to ingest 2,500 calories. For instance, you'd have to eat 39 pounds of Chinese cabbage a day to ingest 2,500 calories!

Terry has achieved amazing weight-loss results by prescribing bulky foods. Here's an example. Mary came to Dr. Shintani more than five years ago. She was forty-five years old and weighed approximately 206 pounds. She had a typical junk food diet and was diabetic. Mary began

High-Bulk Foods

Food	EMI
Cabbage, Chinese	39
Lettuce	39
Celery	32.8
Cucumber	32.8
Radish	32.1
Zucchini	32.1
Lemon	30.4
Eggplant	28.8
Squash	28.8
Endive	27.3
Grapefruit	27.3
Pepper, chili	27.3
Tomato	27.3
Watercress	27.3
Artichoke	26
Cabbage	22.8
Kumquat	22.8
Beans, green	21.9
Asparagus	21
Spinach	21
Watermelon	21
Bamboo shoots	20.2
Cauliflower	20.2
Mushroom	19.5
Turnip	19.5
Cantaloupe	18.2
Melon	18.2
Mustard greens	17.6
Broccoli	17.1
Peach	16.6

High-Bulk Foods

Food	EMI
Pumpkin	16.6
Tangerine	16.1
Bean sprouts, mung	15.6
Orange	15.6
Okra	15.2
Onion, green	15.2
Loquat	14.8
Onion	14.8
Strawberry	14.8
Lychee	14
Carrot	13
Seaweed (konbu)	12.7
Beet	12.7
Cranberry	12.4
Brussels sprout	12.1
Collard	12.1
Seaweed (wakame)	12.1
Ginger	11.9
Grape	11.9
Soybean sprouts	11.9
Apricot	11.4
Pineapple	10.5
Kale	10.3
Oatmeal	9.93
Potato	9.58
Apple	9.42
Blackberry	9.42
Nectarine	9.26
Plum	9.11
Poi	9.11

eating taro, sweet potato, and poi, and after five days Dr. Shintani was able to take her off the 80 units of insulin she had been on for years. She lost over 50 pounds and has kept it off for more than five years. Others lost over 100 pounds by switching from fast foods to a high-bulk diet. A large amount of food stretches the stomach, sending a signal along the vagus nerve to the brain. Terry told me, "We overeat because we eat too little!" He explained that a Big Mac, large fries, and a shake could fail to fill your stomach and leave you hungry. Terry found that it took 3,000 calories of a standard American high-fat diet to become full but only 1,570 calories on a low-energy-density diet. Those who ate the 1,570 calories ate all they wanted to . . . up to 4.1 pounds a day! The high-density, high-fat group ate only 2.76 pounds of food and never felt full but couldn't shed fat! It's remarkable to think you could eat nearly a pound and a half more food a day and expect to lose weight, but that's exactly what happens. Try it. At first you'll swear it's a mistake, but as you look at the scale the next morning you will be amazed. "If you're overweight," Terry says, "it's not because you eat too much. Our study, the Wai'anae Diet, demonstrates that the people ate more food but they still lost weight. We didn't restrict their eating. We let them eat as much as they wanted. You can't ignore the importance of bulk. The bulk is what gives you the stretching that is so important to satiety."

3. SLOWLY DIGESTED CARBOS

Carbohydrates that are digested slowly are far more satiating than fats or refined sugars and can rival proteins in killing hunger. Chewing, tasting, and swallowing are a big part of satisfying your appetite. Slowly digested carbos take the maximum amount of time to do all three. The intestine takes a far longer time breaking them down so that hunger is killed for a longer duration of time. You will find yourself quickly limited as to the amount of these you can eat since your intestine is on overtime, trying to digest them. The chapter "Drop Your Glucose Load" has a complete list ranging from home-cooked black beans to whole oats, barley, and broccoli. Here are some samples.

Slowly Digested Carbos

Soybeans	Butter beans
Peas, dried	Lima beans, baby, frozen
Brown beans	Split peas, yellow, boiled
Barley	Chickpeas
Kidney beans	Barley kernel
Beans, dried	Rye rice
Lentils	Haricot (navy) beans
Green beans	Star pastina, boiled 5 min.
Black beans	Tortillas
Apricots, dried	Pinto beans

Water

A glass of room temperature water at least thirty minutes before a meal helps fill you up and decrease your hunger. But water plays a disastrous role in weight gain when drunk during a meal, especially the ice-cold water served in most restaurants. Water allows you to slop down food without fully chewing it or enjoying it. Ice-cold water also cranks up the production of digestive enzymes, to increase your hunger. Limit what you drink during a meal to a glass of water. For its maximal effect, eat fiber-rich foods before your meal with a glass of water. The fiber will rapidly expand to fill, even bloat you before you sit down for the real meal.

LOW TO HIGH

Make no bones about it. Kids didn't invent the slogan "I'm full" for nothing. Fill yourself with low-density, calorie-poor, super-healthful foods and there just won't be that much room left to cheat. By the time you get to the high-density great-tasting foods, you won't be able to overeat since you'll have a tremendous buffer of gums and fibers to protect you against any dietary indiscretions.

The critical question this section raises is this: Will changes in the composition of the diet to one higher in bulk and fiber lead to weight loss? In other words, can you lose weight simply by changing the composition of the diet rather than eating less food? Ernst Schaefer, M.D., director of the Lipid Metabolism Laboratory at Tufts University School of Medicine recently reported in the *Journal of the American Medical Association* that a high-bulk, high-fiber, low-fat diet does promote weight loss. Participants in his study were able to eat as much as they wanted and lost weight because of the fiber and bulk of the diet. Dr. Schaefer says, "Patients all adjusted downward. One thousand calories of the 15 percent low-fat diet weighed about 1,250 grams. One thousand calories of the average American diet weighed about 900 grams." Patients in his study forced to overeat this diet complained bitterly and, when given a choice, automatically dropped their caloric intake enough to enjoy substantial weight loss.

Dr. Schaefer has a fairly simple prescription for losing weight. He says, "The best way to lower calories is to eat foods that are bulky.

High-fiber foods can be eaten naturally with plenty of fruits and vegetables." Although there is a well-founded fear that a very low-fat diet can actually increase blood fats called triglycerides and make you fatter, those patients in Dr. Schaefer's program actually lowered their triglycerides and lost fat because they ate so much less food. The critical point is that a low-fiber, high refined-flour diet that is low in fat will increase your triglycerides and will make you fat because there's nothing in it to tell you to stop eating. That's why standard low-fat diets make many people fat and cause their triglycerides to soar. Even Vice President Al Gore, who eats a low-fat diet, has triglycerides well above normal . . . just as bad as having a high cholesterol. Dumping the refined flours and adding the fiber and bulk dramatically changes the equation to both lose weight and change your blood fats in a healthy direction.

SATISFY THE BRAIN

Deep in the brain lies an incredibly sophisticated hunger control center in what is termed the hypothalamus. Like a Pentagon communications nerve center, it receives and sorts through myriad different transmissions from the digestive tract, the eyes, tongue, nose, muscles, fat stores, and from foods themselves. For instance, amino acids in proteins and carbohydrates tell the hypothalamus when the body has restocked. There is a direct nerve communication from the stomach when it becomes full. Muscle fuel stores can even signal the brain when they are empty.

The goal is to satisfy the hypothalamus to kill hunger. However, the hypothalamus is very picky. You may max out your craving for sugar, but still have a massive appetite left for fat. Here's an example. When monkeys are hungry, their brain responds to the sight and taste of sugar, but as the monkey consumes the sugar, his brain becomes less responsive to it and the desire for sugar gradually decreases. However, if the monkey was then offered a peanut, his brain responds and the monkey gladly eats the peanut, lusting for fat. The bottom line is that you must deal with all your appetites to succeed in satisfying the brain.

1. PROTEIN FIRST

James Stubbs, Ph.D., of the Rowett Research Institute in Aberdeen, Scotland, proposes that there is a hierarchy in the satiating effects of foods. His work shows that protein is more satiating than carbohydrate, which is more satiating than fat. "From a metabolic viewpoint, the human body is analogous to an engine which continually runs but has a specific order in which it burns up certain fuels since it can store an excess intake of some fuels less readily than others."

There is almost no storage capacity for protein, a limited storage capacity for carbohydrate, and an enormous, almost unlimited storage for fat. Dr. Stubbs's theory holds that the body will quickly say "no!" to eating an excess of protein. If you think about it, when was the last time you had five pieces of salmon steak or half a dozen whole chickens. Your appetite will die long before you're finished.

But what about French fries, onion rings, fried clams, potato chips, and other fat-laden foods? Unfortunately, if you're trying to lose weight, there is nothing in fat that tells your brain to say "no."

Proteins, however, have built into them a signal that tells the brain you're getting enough. Part of that may be to protect the body. Excessive amounts of protein may be dangerous to your kidneys and bones so your body has good reason to limit consumption. To use proteins as a way to curb your appetite, you will need at least 100 calories. Studies have found that small amounts of protein work poorly as a satiator. In experiments, volunteers "preload" with protein — that is, eat protein before other foods are eaten. A high-protein meal produces a greater sensation of fullness and a decreased desire to eat compared to a high-carbohydrate meal with the same number of calories. In one study, obese subjects decreased the number of calories that they ate at the next meal by 19 percent when they ate 155 calories of protein compared to the same amount of carbohydrate. When Dr. Ed Horton, then at the University of Vermont, tried to deliberately overfeed prisoners in a study of weight gain, they could easily wolf down an extra 1,000 calories of fat or carbohydrate but could rarely get beyond an extra 700 calories of protein. The protein produced a greater sensation of fullness and a decreased desire to eat. Dr. James Stubbs concludes that protein appears to be particularly satiating when given at moderate and large amounts as part of a weight-reducing diet . . . a point not lost on the diet trade. The initial successes of liquid protein diets and Dr. Atkins's diet give credit to this special satiating property of proteins. However, the addition of fats to the Atkins diet and simple sugars to the liquid diet can make them terribly unhealthy ways to lose weight. The protein supplement Met Rx has recently gained huge popularity because of its potential effects as a high-protein weight-loss remedy. Be warned that some studies fed their subjects unrealistically high amounts of protein, over 60 percent of a meal. To avoid the potential long-term dangers of super-high-protein diets, there is another solution. Eat protein as the first part of your meal, let it digest to the point that it has time to signal the brain, then resume your meal. For good reason, that's the opposite of the way most meals are presented in restaurants, which wouldn't be able to sell more than two courses if they filled you up with protein first. The conventional meal is built to stimulate the appetite and to leave room for other foods . . . just exactly what you don't want. It's a great reason to start breakfast and lunch with a good protein load. A glass of milk, a black bean soup, or your main fish or meat course as starters is the way to go. It has a wonderful lasting effect. Harvard's Dr. George Blackburn has long recommended drinking a glass of skim milk before any meal. "Milk is the secret ingredient, fortified with vitamins and minerals, which is why people feel so good. It will satiate you and you'll be able to cut back so easily on 20 percent of portions," says Dr. Blackburn.

Dr. Judith Wurtman has just completed a study that shows the value of eating protein early in the day. She found that the more successful dieters consumed more protein in the morning and most of their carbohydrates in the late afternoon and early evening. Dieters who flipped the pattern and ate more carbos in the morning, then protein in the afternoon, overate.

The emphasis on protein may seem to fly in the face of conventional wisdom that we already eat too much protein. But let's look for a moment at what I call the pasta junkie. That person may indeed get protein in the pastas and breads and cereals that he eats, but he's not getting the concentrated "hit" of protein needed for its satiating effect. The "food brakes" in pasta just aren't strong enough. Pasta doesn't have enough fiber or slowly digested carbos to kill hunger, and it doesn't have enough protein to satiate either. The solution is to back off the extra carbos and to consume more concentrated protein as skim milk, beans, fish, and fowl. By strategically eating protein to cut hunger, you'll cut your total calories.

2. CUT THE CRAVING FOR FAT

Galanin is a brain hormone that regulates the body's desire for fat. As galanin levels rise, so does your desire to eat foods that contain fat. Sarah Leibowitz of The Rockefeller University showed that when galanin is injected into the hypothalamus of laboratory animals, they select more fatty foods. Even worse, the more galanin you make, the more fat you store, so it's critical to make less galanin by eating less fat. Here's how:

Grazing

One way to lower levels of galanin is through snacking. Here's why. Galanin is released when the body breaks down body fat, as it does during dieting or when several hours have passed between meals. When the body breaks down body fat, fat particles are released into the blood that travel to the hypothalamus and trigger galanin's release. But if you graze rather than eat three big meals or diet, you'll seriously cut your craving for fat by dropping galanin production. Robert Pritikin has also found that grazing works wonders for serious compulsive eaters. "You just eat all the time. The frequent feedings minimize gorging because you just ate," says Robert. At the Pritikin Longevity Center in Santa Monica, California, guests eat three meals plus snacks at 10:30 and 2:30. Eating less fat also drops galanin production. Humans didn't start eating three meals a day until the Industrial Revolution. According to Stephen Bailey, Ph.D., a Tufts University professor of anthropology, the "three squares a day" evolved to fit with factory life. "If you look back in time, people grazed. That's what our bodies are meant to do," says Dr. Bailey. But modern man has created this sense that snacking is somehow inappropriate. Do you ever remember your dentist or pediatrician saying: Now be sure to snack between meals? Dr. Bailey says, "If you snack you don't ever feel as hungry when you sit down to eat a 'meal.' As a result, you won't overeat. The norm today is that we fast between meals and suffer the consequences. When we sit down to eat a meal our stomachs are empty, we eat rapidly, and we eat a great deal. We eat so quickly," says Dr. Bailey, "we don't have time for the foods we eat to send hormonal signals to the brain that we have plenty of food in our stomach. Three squares condition your body to make every meal a major opportunity to gain weight. Your body slows down its metabolic rate and increases its efficiency at storing calories between meals, so that it can gorge during meals. Studies show you will gain more weight if you have the same number of calories and eat only one meal as opposed to distributing those same calories over four meals."

Many dieters have such a mortal fear of food that they confine themselves to just one or two meals a day . . . with disastrous results. Dr. Bailey, with the School of Nutrition at Tufts, studied students who relied on only two meals a day. "Basically they spend large periods of the day fasting, only eating a light late coffee-and-bagel breakfast and an enormous, high-calorie, late dinner between 7 and 9 at night." Fasting had negative effects on their cognitive ability and disastrous effects on the waistline as judged by the ten- to twenty-pound weight gain.

If you snack and eat small meals you will never experience that type of ravishing hunger that most Americans erroneously describe as merely being hungry. Think about that for a moment. What we perceive as hunger is a much more profound symptom than we recognize because we have trained ourselves to wait for hunger, to endure hunger, to enjoy hunger.

Are humans made to nibble? Dr. Bailey says that our nearest genetic cousins are primates who don't have meals. Rather, they eat and sleep continuously. You can't define mealtime for chimps. "That, combined with historical evidence that meals are structured around the imperatives of factory life, suggests that the whole notion of meals is an artificial and recent construct," he says. Also, all over the world, young kids, who are not yet "socialized" into eating three meals a day, tend to snack naturally, another indicator that the three meal construct is unnatural.

Historical data indicates that the Farming Model of eating was the way people really ate. You got up before dawn, had a small meal, worked for a while, had another meal, worked for a while more, had a big midday meal, worked until it was pretty late, had a snack, had a supper much later, and then you went to sleep. The only big meal was at midday, giving you the opportunity to work it off.

The public has badly misinterpreted the meaning of snacking to include mostly junk, refined carbos. A snack should be a small meal complete with protein and hard carbos. By eliminating protein and fiber, you have eliminated appetite control.

Dr. David Jenkins says, "I think it's very beneficial for people to snack if they can remember that they've snacked and not go on to eat full meals as well." The big trick is to become satisfied with smaller meals, realizing that you really are satisfied and needn't continue to eat. You have the added carrot of knowing that your next food is never more than several hours away.

Eat Less Fat

The more fat you eat, the more galanin you make and the more fat you crave. Eating fat becomes a real catch-22. Dr. Leibowitz showed that those rats that ate diets that were more than 40 percent fat had twice as much galanin in a certain part of the hypothalamus than did the rats that ate a diet that contained less than 20 percent fat. This is how a high-fat diet fundamentally changes the brain into a fat-craving machine. By creating less galanin, you'll eat less fat. The brain feels best with a diet around 15 to 20 percent fat.

Jack Wilmore, M.D., of the University of Texas at Austin, says, "I'm concerned about fat in the diet because no matter what kind of fat you have in the diet, it's a stimulant to eat more calories than you normally would if you didn't have the fat in your diet. Remember the old potato chip advertisement: 'Bet you can't just eat one?' Food manufacturers have known that for years. It's a palatability issue. The more palatable, the more of it we eat." Galanin release may also be cut off by eating more protein. I'm impressed that really lean people instinctively order high-protein meals. That may take a little bit of willpower in the ordering process, but once you start your protein course, your desire for fat will decrease. Since galanin production naturally rises through the late morning into the afternoon, you can employ an easy strategy to beat your fat cravings.

- Stay away from fats in the morning when you won't have much natural craving for fats.
- Avoid fat at lunch, the worst meal to eat fat because your brain is nearing its natural peak production of galanin to which eating fat will add an extra production run to create sky-high galanin levels.
- Eat a high-protein breakfast, lunch, and midafternoon snack to cut the production of galanin.

Lower Your Insulin

A rock-steady insulin level is key to decreasing the craving for fat since a fall in insulin level also stimulates more galanin production. The next chapters tell you how.

Avoid Fat/Sugar Combinations

It's hard to really overdose on pure fat or pure sugar. Here's why: Plain fat doesn't have any taste at all. It's only by flavoring fat that it becomes palatable. And too much sugar does make a drink or dessert way too sweet. But by adding fat to sugar you have a fatal combination. You first make the fat taste good, then you can crank up the amount of sugar to 70 percent without making the food taste too sweet. This way you overeat sweets and fats. The other element that fat adds is texture or mouth feel. Food marketing people like to say that foods have to have "taste, taste, taste." What they really mean, according to food scientists, is "fat, fat, fat." The addition of sugar to a high-fat diet is the most dangerous combination of all for sustained weight gain.

3. SATISFY YOUR CARBOHYDRATE HUNGER

Carbohydrates are the most dangerous foods for the brain to crave since you can eat them even more endlessly than fat. The most common mistake is to eat quickly digested junk carbos that cause the most intense craving for more carbos. The only practical means of killing the craving for carbohydrate is to eat slowly digested carbos, such as beans, since those make only a modest increase in blood sugar. Judith Wurtman, Ph.D., maintains that carbohydrate cravings can be satisfied with any carbohydrate. She says, "The only discipline that has to be used is to satisfy them with foods that do little caloric damage and have nutritional value." That means slowly digested carbos. "Real cravings should be recognized in relation to stress and satisfied with a 'dose' of carbohydrate that has a pharmacologic effect on the brain, is fat free, and should be eaten on a relatively empty stomach so it's digested quickly so that other foods do not interfere. You can prevent cravings that cause you to eat impulsively and out of control by acknowledging that you need the carbohydrates at a certain time of day, usually late afternoon, and eating enough hard carbos to satisfy that appetite. You can also carbo load for stressful situations."

4. SATIATE ALL YOUR HUNGERS

Satiety is not general, but is specific to particular foods that you consume. As the pleasantness of one food declines as you eat more of it, other uneaten foods remain quite attractive to the sight and the taste. That builds a natural tendency to switch from food to food to maintain palatability. That's why you can plow through an amazing number of calories when presented with hors d'oeuvres circulated at a cocktail party. Different hungers are critical to survival because the consumption of a variety of foods is essential to capture all of the nutrients that the body requires. But to maintain perfect weight control, you must be wary that this is a trap that will lead you from one fattening food to another. Barbara Rolls, Ph.D., of Pennsylvania State University, found a great enhancement of intake when four successive courses of very different foods were presented. In a four-course meal of sausages, bread and butter, chocolate whipped dessert, and bananas, intake was 60 percent more than when just one of the foods was presented. So, the greater the differences between foods, the greater the enhancement of intake. Dr. Rolls's principles of hunger enhancement show a very quick way to become big as a horse, but the following suggestions will help you cut your craving.

Food Substitution

Foods with similar sensory properties but differing calorie counts are equally effective at cutting your hunger. So as long as you know what hungers you have to satisfy, you can eat foods that are far less fattening, even thinning, to fill you up. For instance, coconut cream pie and cantaloupe both fit into the same sensory experience, but with vastly different caloric and health properties. Consumption of either sweet food can decrease the hunger for other foods with similar sensory properties. So if you're really swaying toward the cream pie, dig into the melon. Within minutes, your lust for the pie will be severely damped. Curiously, it appears to be the sensory properties of the foods and not their composition that signals the brain. That means you could have an extremely healthy tortilla and bean dish and get the same satiety as a high-fat fish and chips.

Eat Good Foods First

The decreases in the pleasantness of a specific food occur very rapidly after eating, within two minutes, and decline in magnitude over the following hour. So satisfy yourself with good, wholesome food first. If you crave a fat or sugary food, savor the first bite and your urge should subside.

5. ABSTINENCE

Alcoholics Anonymous long ago found that if an alcoholic continued to tempt himself with the taste of alcohol, he would fail. The New Hampshire chapter of Overeaters Anonymous has undertaken a similar theme with food. Sure, you can try to modify your cravings but you're still playing with fire. They have found great success in abstaining by following advice embedded in their motto: no fat, no sugar.

6. A LOW INSULIN LEVEL

Dr. Judith Rodin's research, while she was a professor of psychology and psychiatry at Yale University, showed that people are hungriest and like sweet tastes more when insulin levels are high. Here's why. When people snack on sugary foods, their insulin level rises. The insulin stimulates the appetite, causes repeated sugar cravings, and results in people eating more food and calories at the next meal than do people who snack on other foods or drink water. There's even a breed of "hyperresponders" whose insulin level jumps at the sight or smell of food. By maintaining a low insulin level you don't create the general dysphoria that follows a sugar high and creates the craving for carbohydrates and sweets. The next chapter tells you how.

7. SMALL DOSES

This is the neatest single food as drug trick in the book, giving your brain the endorphin buzz it wants, with just a small dose of chocolate. Here's how it works. Put a piece of chocolate in your mouth. The aroma of the chocolate is pumped up behind your palette into your nasal cavity by swallowing and chewing. Your nose picks up the aroma by a process called retro nasal olfaction. This triggers the brain to make endorphins to reward you for eating the chocolate. Scientists call this a hard-wired response, by which they mean there is a direct "hot line" from the mouth to the brain that completely bypasses the stomach. Paul Rozin, Ph.D., professor at the University of Pennsylvania, found that "the oral experience reduces the craving for chocolate. From our study, we infer that the single most potent thing is the actual texture and aroma. . . . We gave participants chocolate in a capsule and it did nothing for their craving."

If you ate the chocolate on an empty stomach, you would have the blood sugar and insulin surge that might cause you to eat the whole box. But if you slowly suck on just one or two pieces after filling your stomach with high-fiber foods, there won't be any surge in blood sugar or insulin and you will still get the endorphin surge without having to wait for all your food to digest. That way a very modest amount of sweets will satisfy you. So just like your mom said, reward yourself for a meal well eaten. But remember that you don't need a huge gooey dessert to get the hit you're looking for. The after-dinner mint was a lot smarter idea than most of us have given it credit for.

8. CHEW GUM

Keep the sweet taste in your mouth and use the repetitive motion of chewing to build more serotonin in your brain.

9. MONOTONY

When Michael Crichton writes a new bestseller, he chooses to eat the same lunch every single day. There are several excellent reasons for doing so. First, it saves an enormous amount of time struggling with choosing what to eat or, even worse, developing new recipes and shopping lists. Second, once you have the perfectly engineered lunch, you know exactly what it will do for you. If you have a big dinosaur escape scene coming up, you don't want to find yourself suddenly lacking in strength or resolve. But the most important reason is that you can carefully control your intake. I'll have the same lunch for a month or more in a row. I know I'll be satisfied, so there's no need to down extra calories. You'll also find that this approach works for you in giving you the quickly sated quality that Aristotle was looking for. Unexpected new tastes can cause you to splurge, but a familiar yet still tasty lunch really kills your hunger pretty quickly and predictably. While writing this book I ate a whole wheat quesadilla with black beans every lunch for five months. I'm full until nighttime and don't need to eat much more than a midafternoon snack and before-bed snack. Curiously, it's monotony that allows most of the world to keep their appetite in check. They eat the same rice and beans every day, year in year out. Our tremendous diversity of foods allows us a never-ending range of dietary sins. The diets of traditional peoples are monotonous. While we have this notion that breakfast has to be very different from dinner, many societies serve dinner leftovers for breakfast — for instance, beans for breakfast, lunch, and dinner.

10. PREEMPTIVE EATING

When you deliberately fill yourself in advance of hunger, you immunize yourself from the sight, smell, even taste of food. The old axiom that you shouldn't go shopping while you're hungry derives from the fact that just the appearance of food in the supermarket can cause you to overshop for the wrong kinds of foods. In a later chapter, "Feedforward Eating," I'll develop a complete preemptive eating plan for you.

11. SOBRIETY

Professor Angelo Tremblay of Laval University conducted research that will disappoint beer drinkers around the world. The brain doesn't register the calories in alcohol. Whatever diet you are eating, alcohol adds extra calories without depressing your appetite at all. In the Quebec study, researchers studied 351 men and 360 women and found that beer drinking did not cut down the appetite. Alcohol constitutes 5 to 7 percent of the daily caloric intake of American men, less in women.

Drop Your Glucose Load

Carbo loading gained great popularity in the 1980s as a way for elite marathoners to run harder longer. Never in the history of nutrition has a good idea gone so wrong. Now most of America carbo loads every day at every meal. Sure, several hundred world-class marathoners benefited by crossing the finish line a few minutes faster, but tens of millions of carbo-overloaded Americans made their way into the history books as the fattest generation ever.

Conventional Wisdom
Eat all the carbos you want.

LEAN
Cut your glucose load.

ROAD MAP

This chapter introduces the premier concept in nutrition today, glucose overload, the emerging number-one cause of dangerous obesity. If there is only one single point that you take home from this book, it is that decreasing your glucose load is the most effective way of becoming lean and controlling your weight. You'll find many methods of lowering your glucose load as well as an extensive list of low glucose load foods. Since the danger of a high glucose load comes from the high insulin level that results, you'll find additional measures to decrease your insulin level.

GLUCOSE OVERLOAD

Glucose load is a measure of the total amount of glucose that passes through our bloodstreams in a day. Think of thousands of cars crammed onto a California freeway at rush hour choking the flow of traffic. One high-glucose meal after the other puts an incredible strain on the highway system of blood vessels that course through our bodies by cramming it full of glucose. What's glucose? Glucose is the body's chief source of energy. It is a simple sugar that passes easily into the bloodstream from the digestive tract when we eat carbohydrates. Virtually all carbohydrates can ultimately be broken down into glucose, their lowest common denominator. The term "blood sugar" is actually slang for blood glucose, which is the concentration of glucose in the blood.

The reason this concept is so important is that we tend to think that only candy bars, ice cream, and other sugary foods affect blood glucose levels. In fact, every carbohydrate you eat, from breakfast cereals, pastas, and breads to LifeSavers and soft drinks, has the same end result: higher levels of glucose in the bloodstream. The exceptions are some fruits, which end up largely as fructose and have little effect on blood sugar levels.

You might say, "Hey, I don't eat that much sugar." Hear this. Sugar consumption in America during the past 150 years has skyrocketed. In 1840 our forebears consumed four teaspoons of sweeteners daily. Today, the USDA estimates that the average American consumes almost a cup of sugar a day. Smart weight-conscious Americans may believe that they successfully avoid these sugary foods, and that's the trap. These savvy consumers eat hundreds of foods that rapidly convert into glucose. Surprisingly, most of them are the highly overpromoted "complex carbohydrates." You see, complex carbos are far from equal. Sure, whole grains are terrific, but white flour pasta, breads, cereals, bagels, and pancakes all earn the title "complex carbos" and are even labeled "low-fat" foods. Though these carbohydrates are indeed complex because they are made up of enormous sugar molecules instead of tiny "simple" sugars, they quickly break down into glucose once they are digested in the body. This causes a large and sustained increase in blood sugar. When you sum up the total of all the glucose produced by a day's worth of carbohydrates, you arrive at what researchers call your total glucose load. Here's how it works.

DETERMINING GLUCOSE LOAD

After eating a food on an empty stomach, blood sugar is measured at regular intervals until a peak level is detected. Dr. David Jenkins of the University of Toronto and other researchers made this measurement for hundreds of foods. Each carbohydrate was assigned a glucose value on a scale that ranges from a low of 0 to a high of over 100. (Nutrition aficionados use the term "GI," while researchers use the term "glycemic index.") Carbohydrates low on that index, such as beans, generate a very small rise in blood sugar after they are eaten. That puts an insignificant "load" on your system. Foods with a high-glucose index, from instant mashed potatoes and white bread, Twinkies and muffins, to bagels, are digested very quickly, giving rise to high blood sugars and placing a heavy "load" on your body. Since these high-glucose foods are basically glucose bombs, the more of these foods in your diet, the higher your "glucose load." These high-glucose carbos, composed of thousands of glucose molecules strung together, enter your body like a Trojan horse. Since they don't taste sweet or look sweet, we eat tons of them . . . falsely believing that they are healthy for us. But once your digestive tract strips their disguise by breaking them apart, millions of glucose molecules flow freely into your bloodstream like water through a broken dike. The more of those glucose molecules that enter your system during a day, the higher your glucose load. What troubles the nation's leading nutritionists is that you need not have outrageously high-glucose foods to have a high glucose load. Foods with a moderate glucose index, such as white rice or pasta, can give you a sky-high glucose load if you eat even a moderate amount. While individual foods that cause large rises in blood sugar are said to have a high glucose index, an entire meal, built on foods with a high or even medium glucose index, is said to have a high glucose load.

Since these tests are run on different people under different conditions, these values are good to within plus or minus 10 points. You should therefore look at them for their relative value. For example, rice bran is listed as being one point higher than soybeans. On any given day one could measure higher than the other. However, you can count on the fact that they are both very low-glucose foods.

HOW GLUCOSE OVERLOAD MAKES YOU FAT

The emerging supervillain of overweight people around the world is an excess of the hormone insulin. Think that's overstated? What could be worse than a hormone that makes you fat, stresses you out, clogs your arteries, raises your blood pressure, increases your risk of cancer, speeds up the aging process, leads to diabetes, and breeds heart attacks? Insulin does all that in spades. Excess insulin is the most likely reason that you are overweight and the biggest reason that those extra pounds will kill you. Insulin is the kingpin that switches your body's weight-gaining functions into high gear and is the hormone most responsible for the ballooning of America. How? Too much insulin jam-packs fat cells with fats, slams the door, and throws away the key. What's the link between glucose load and insulin? The higher your glucose load, the higher your insulin level, because it is glucose load that drives insulin. Here's a brief primer.

You may say, "Hey, I thought you had to have insulin, I never heard it was bad before." True, your body couldn't survive without insulin since its most important role is to rein in high levels of blood sugar. Your body sees a rising blood sugar level as a life-threatening danger that it has to vigorously defend against. Why? A normal blood sugar level is around 60 to 120. Very high levels, say 800 or so, can lead to coma. If your blood sugar is moderately high over a prolonged period of time, it can lead to loss of vision, kidney disease, heart disease, even blindness. Given this extreme degree of danger, your body will do whatever it can to keep blood glucose within bounds. If blood glucose rises quickly, after your body is hit with a high glucose load, your body blows out huge amounts of insulin into your bloodstream, like an elite fire brigade spraying fire retardant foam onto a flash fire. This is called an insulin surge. Every single time glucose gushes into your bloodstream, you set off the alarm to pour out the insulin. The response time is a lot faster than your average 911 call, taking just one to two minutes. The most powerful way to jettison excess sugar is to find a dumping ground. You guessed it. That dumping ground is the vast wasteland known as body fat with its enormous capacity to soak up excess calories. The more excess glucose you dump into your body, the more insulin acts to dump it into the extra pounds of fat that form around your midsection. Insulin is up to thirty times more effective at moving extra calories into fat than into muscle, making it an effective superstuffer of fat cells. The more fat you eat, the further those floodgates swing open. That's why the combination of fat and high-glucose foods is so incredibly fattening.

Your doctor may disagree about the danger of glucose load. He or she is in good company. The diabetes community has pooh-poohed the idea of the glucose index for many years. So has the obesity community. But all of that has changed, and here's why. A just published work by the Department of Nutrition at the Harvard School of Public Health shows that the higher your glucose load, the higher your risk of diabetes is likely to be. And that can mean sky-high insulin. This classic study of over 90,000 health-care professionals for the first time ever shows that the effect of glucose load is big enough to be seen across the entire population. That means that everyone responds poorly to a high glucose load, some just worse than others.

You don't have to be Claus von Bulow to know that high levels of insulin are dangerous. The extent of its effect is truly staggering — from increased risk of heart disease and cancer to a higher cholesterol, more stress, kidney failure, and diabetes.

FOODS THAT CAUSE GLUCOSE OVERLOAD
HIGH-GLUCOSE CARBOS

Carbos are the primary food that raise your glucose load, but you will find that carbos are far from equal. High-glucose carbos cause the largest increase in your blood sugar and insulin levels. You should eat an extremely limited number of these. I use them only for flavoring low-GI foods. There are some real surprises on this list, such as bagels, cream of wheat, instant rice, and potatoes. If you're really trying to lose weight, wipe these foods off your grocery list. The higher the number in the following table, the higher your blood sugar level will

High-Glucose Carbohydrates

Food	Glucose Index
Hamburger bun	61
Ice cream	61
Avon, canned	61
New potato	62
Semolina	64
Shortbread	64
Raisins	64
Macaroni and cheese, boxed	64
Beetroot	64
Flan	65
Oat kernel	65
Rye flour	65
Couscous	65
High-fiber rye crispbread	65
Sucrose	65
Cream of Wheat (cereal)	66
Life (cereal)	66
Museli (cereal)	66
Arrowroot	66
Pineapple	66
Angel food	67
Croissant	67
Grapenuts (cereal)	67
Puffed Wheat (cereal)	67
Breton wheat cracker	67
Stoned Wheat Thins	67
Soft drink, Fanta	68
Maize, cornmeal	68
Mars Bar	68
Crumpet	69
Wheat bread, gluten free	69
Shredded Wheat	69
Melba toast	70
Wheat biscuit	70
Potato, white, mashed	70
LifeSavers	70
Fruit, dried	70
Golden Grahams (crackers)	71
Millet	71
Carrot	71
Bagel, white	72
Water crackers	72

High-Glucose Carbohydrates

Food	Glucose Index
Watermelon	72
Rutabaga	72
Popcorn	72
Kaiser rolls	73
Potato, boiled, mashed	73
Corn chips	73
Honey	73
Bread stuffing	74
Cheerios (cereal)	74
French fries	75
Pumpkin	75
Donut	76
Waffle	76
Cocoapops (cereal)	77
Vanilla wafers	77
Broad beans	79
Grapenut Flakes (cereal)	80
Jelly beans	80
Puffed crispbread	81
Rice Krispies (cereal)	82
Rice cake	82
Corn Chex (cereal)	83
Potato, instant	83
Corn Flakes (cereal)	84
Potato, baked	85
Crispix	87
Rice, instant	87
Rice, white, low amylose	88
Rice Chex (cereal)	89
Cactus jam	91
Rice pasta, brown	92
French baguette	95
Rockmelon	95
Parsnip	97
Glucose tablets	102
Maltose	105
Tofu frozen dessert, nondairy	115

Table adapted with permission from the *American Journal of Clinical Nutrition* 62 (1995): 871–935.

rise after you eat them! If you really love these foods, mix them with extremely low-GI foods . . . once you've lost the weight you want to. An example would be low-GI soybeans mixed with high-GI rice, which averages out to a moderate glucose load.

An excess of glucose makes most women and many men sleepier than they otherwise would be. Our predecessors ruined their afternoon's work with two-martini lunches; we cut our ability to put in a strong afternoon and evening of work with a glucose overload.

MODERATE-GLUCOSE CARBOS

Medium-GI foods should be eaten in limited quantities. If you are really trying to lose weight, eliminate them altogether. While a high-fiber content makes oat bran, oatmeal, and bulgur exceptions, the majority — from macaroni, rice, noodles to potato crisps and spaghetti — will make you fat. Walter Willett, M.D., Dr.P.H., the Frederick John Stare professor of epidemiology and nutrition and the chairman of the department of nutrition at the Harvard School of Public Health, told me that the real surprise was how much medium-glucose carbos added to the glucose load. They appear to be safe and conventional, but eaten in moderate to large quantities they will make you fat. The higher the food's glucose index, the higher your blood sugar will be after eating them. A diet full of them will keep you hungry. Just think of how hungry you are after a meal of Chinese takeout which is heavy on rice and noodles. The food literally washes through your system too fast to keep you satisfied for long.

At this point, you would be justified in saying, "Gee, all those grains, breads, and cereals I thought were great are trash." Are *any* grains good for you? There is a radical theory that says no! Here's how it goes: After the development of methodical planting and harvesting of grains, there was a dramatic decrease in human health. According to Stephen Bailey, Ph.D., an anthropologist at Tufts University, "In places where you see a transition from hunting and gathering to an actual reliance on domesticated foods, you get a shortening of life-span, you get evidence of episodes of malnutrition or undernutrition in childhood, and people become physically smaller. It's pretty clear. There's evidence in the skeletons. There is also an increase in certain

Moderate-Glucose Carbos

Food	Glucose Index
Capellini	45
Macaroni, boiled 5 minutes	45
Romano beans	46
Linguine, thick durum	46
Lactose	46
Fruit loaf, wheat with dried fruit	47
Instant noodles	47
Bulgur	48
Baked beans	48
Green peas	48
Corn, high amylose	49
Chocolate	49
Rye kernel	50
Ice cream, low fat	50
Tortellini cheese	50
Yam	51
Kiwifruit	52
Banana	53
Pound sponge cake	54
Special K (cereal)	54
Buckwheat	54
Sweet potato	54
Potato crisps	54
Linseed rye	55

Moderate-Glucose Carbos

Food	Glucose Index
Oatmeal	55
Rich tea biscuit	55
Fruit cocktail, canned	55
Mango	55
Spaghetti, durum	55
Sweet corn	55
Sultanas	56
Pontiac, boiled	56
Potato, white	56
Pita, white	57
Orange juice	57
Bran Chex (cereal)	58
Peach, canned, heavy syrup	58
Rice vermicelli	58
Blueberry	59
Pastry	59
Rice, white, high amylose	59
Digestive biscuits	59
Bran	60
Pizza, cheese	60

Table adapted with permission from the *American Journal of Clinical Nutrition* 62 (1995): 871–935.

kinds of the diseases that actually leave a record in the bone. This is a general pattern that we see."

Our ancestors were far taller at the end of the Stone Age than now. What does that have to do with health? Bob Fogel, a recent Nobel laureate in economics, determined that height is a real indicator of well-being. The taller, the healthier and wealthier. What grains did was to displace the fresh vegetables that Stone Age man ate with nutritionally inferior carbos. Nutritionally inferior you say? To prove it, look at the nutritional values for vegetables (in chapter 13), which score a high of 461 points. Then look at the very highest ranked grain (in chapter 11), which ranks a measly 73. Replacing veggies with grains caused an enormous loss of nutrients. But even worse, the beginning of modern agriculture rapidly increased the glucose load of the human diet with the addition of grains. Can man adapt to a high glucose load? Over two million years, there has been the most minute shift in human genes. In the eight thousand years since the agricultural revolution, not even a second's sweep has gone by on the genetic clock . . . too little time for genes to mutate. When you use the long lens of time as a judge and look at the human body to see what it was designed to do, it was designed to eat low-glucose carbos.

SATURATED FATS

Saturated fats change the outer layer of your muscle, called the membrane. A normal muscle membrane lets sugar flow through it easily. Eating large amounts of saturated fats and some polyunsaturated fats makes your muscle far more resistant to the effects of insulin, allowing your blood sugar to rise, which increases your glucose load.

SATURATED FATS AND HIGH-GLUCOSE CARBOS

If saturated fats cause a higher glucose load and high-glucose carbos cause a high glucose load, you'd expect that the two added together would be bad news . . . and you'd be right! You have a real two plus two equals ten condition. Dr. James Barnard of UCLA and the Pritikin Longevity Center found out why. In laboratory rats, fat alone could not make the animals enormously fat; it took the addition of sugar to light the fuse. Some fuse! Rats given the combination of 40 percent fat and 40 percent sugar grew fatter than those ingesting any other combination of foods. Jim has made the same observation in people. "It really isn't how much food you eat, it's what kind, and the high-fat, high-sugar combination is the worst of all." He's confirmed what overweight people have said for years: They don't eat very much food. In fact, Jim was most struck by how as his overweight subjects ate less and less, they still gained weight; if they stuck to the fat, sugar combination, they were doomed to stay fat. Now almost no human being eats a fat and sugar diet, but we do eat those high-glucose carbohydrates that quickly run up blood sugar levels in combination with fats.

Examples:
- Fried dough
- Bagel with cream cheese
- Fried rice
- Ice cream sundae
- Pastries

HIGH BODY FAT

As your body fat rises, so does your glucose load. That's because your insulin becomes less and less effective as you become more and more overweight. With each additional pound, large amounts of glucose remain in the blood, increasing your glucose load. If you are genetically predisposed to diabetes, you become even more insulin resistant for each extra pound of fat you carry.

BIG MEALS

Big meals are death. If you have to eat for a living, entertaining guests at big dinners, you may be doomed. A big load of food at any given meal will spike your insulin, big time. There's no worse time than evening, when a big load of insulin will load up your arteries and fat cells all night long. Naturally if your meal is made up of high-glucose carbos, fats, and easily digested proteins, you could achieve a new personal record. A major steak with instant mashed potatoes, the jet fuel of the fast-burning carbos, will make your insulin soar through the stratosphere into the wee hours. Don't confuse a big-calorie meal with a high-volume meal. You can eat a large meal of high-bulk, high-fiber foods without bumping your insulin.

HOW TO LOWER YOUR GLUCOSE LOAD
LOW-GLUCOSE CARBOS

You may literally eat all the low-GI carbos you want because they are so filling and have such a small effect on glucose load. Examples are beans, cruciferous vegetables, and high-fiber, low-sugar cereals. The foods with the lowest numbers in the list that follows have the lowest glucose loads.

Low-Glucose Carbos

Food	Glucose Index
Nopal, prickly pear cactus	7
Yogurt, low-fat, unsweetened, plain	14
Acorns, stewed, with venison	16
Soybeans	18
Rice bran	19
Cherries	22
Peas, dried	22
Plum	24
Barley	25
Grapefruit	25
Mesquite cake	25
Kidney beans	27
Peach, fresh	28
Beans, dried	29
Lentils	29
Yellow tepary bean broth	29
Green beans	30
Black beans	30
Apricot, dried	31
Butter beans	31
Skim milk	32
Lima beans, baby, frozen	32
Split peas, yellow, boiled	32

Low-Glucose Carbos

Food	Glucose Index
Chickpeas	33
Rye rice	34
Apple	36
Pear	36
Spaghetti, whole wheat	37
Haricot (navy) beans	38
Star pastina, boiled 5 min.	38
Tomato	38
Tortilla	38
Brown beans	38
Pinto beans	39
Corn hominy	40
All Bran	42
Black-eyed beans	42
Grapes	43
Orange	43
Spirali, durum	43
Mixed grain	45

Table adapted with permission from the *American Journal of Clinical Nutrition* 62 (1995): 871–935.

While white flour pastas have a medium glycemic index, whole wheat pastas are in the low-GI category because they are higher in fiber and low in refined flour. Low-glucose carbos also drop your insulin level. Clients at the Pritikin Longevity Center in Santa Monica, California, achieve large drops in insulin by eating carbohydrates in their "very unrefined state." The average fasting insulin falls 25 to 30 percent. Low-glucose carbos are very satiating as well, so you will naturally eat fewer carbos, which will cut your glucose load.

MORE VEGETABLE FAT

In the mammoth Harvard Nurses Study, the higher the vegetable fat content of the diet, the lower the risk of running a high insulin level. This is a function of replacing high-glucose carbos with healthy vegetable fats since they have no direct effect on insulin. The health-iest vegetable fats have a high amount of monounsaturated fats, which increase your good cholesterol.

In this way you are changing the composition of your diet to eat less glucose. The table below shows you the relative advantages of vegetable oils. Those with the most monounsaturated fats and least saturated fats are rated the highest. To be clear, replacing medium- and high-glucose foods with monounsaturated fats such as olive oil goes a long way to decreasing your glucose load.

MORE PROTEIN

Glucagon is the hormone that sits on the opposite end of the seesaw from insulin, i.e., the higher your glucagon, the lower your insulin. Barry Sears, Ph.D., author of *The Zone,* suggests that by eating more protein, you increase glucagon levels, lowering insulin levels. When a meal is stripped of carbohydrate and only the protein remains, insulin levels rise very little. Protein also helps to kill hunger and energize the brain while keeping insulin levels low. By replacing carbohydrate in a meal with protein, you also decrease your glucose load. Dr. Jacqueline Hart of Beth Israel Deaconess Medical Center in Boston found that a 20 percent protein diet cut glucose load enough to drop the level of fats called triglycerides that result from a high glucose load.

Fatty Acid Composition of Principal Oils

Oil or fat	Saturated (%)	Monounsaturated (%)	Polyunsaturated (%)
Canola oil	6	62	32
High oleic safflower oil	7	80	12
High oleic sunflower oil	8	81	9
Safflower oil	9	13	78
Sunflower oil	12	19	69
Corn oil	13	28	57
Peanut oil	14	50	32
Soybean oil	15	24	61
Olive oil	17	72	11

MORE SOLUBLE FIBER

The Harvard School of Public Health has demonstrated that the higher your overall fiber intake, the lower your risk of running a high insulin level. Dr. Ed Horton says: "There's no question that high fiber can smooth out the glycemic curve." Components of soluble fiber such as guars and pectins form a gummy gel that lines the intestine and slows absorption, blunting the uptake of glucose and decreasing the insulin response. Soluble fibers are so powerful that even if you add sugars to high-fiber foods, your blood sugar rise is still blunted. University of Kentucky's Dr. James W. Anderson was one of the earliest to use gums and guars, agents that slow the digestion of food, with his patients. Even after forty-two months of outpatient followup, Dr. Anderson's patients maintained an average 15-pound weight loss.

FAT LOSS

Losing fat is a case of the thin getting thinner. Here's why. The less fat you have, the better your insulin works and the less insulin you make. In the past, many dieters got stuck because they used heavy concentrations of sugars that boosted insulin levels. Liquid diets, pasta diets, and frozen dinners of high-glucose carbos were prime examples. They locked fat in the cells. By losing fat and maintaining lower insulin levels, you'll turn on the body's fat-burning switches. You may say, "Hey that sounds crazy! How can you tell me to lose fat when that's just what I'm trying to do?" As you shed fat you "get over the hump" and drop enough fat to allow natural fat burning to kick in. When you are thinner, the brain releases key weight control hormones that dramatically cut your craving for carbohydrates and kill your hunger.

LOW GLUCOSE LOAD DIETS

The question I'm most frequently asked about nutrition is this: How can diets that appear to be so vastly different, such as those of Dr. Atkins, Dr. Sears, Dr. Ornish, and Overeaters Anonymous all achieve substantial weight loss? Here's where Perfect Weight Control cuts through. What these doctors and groups hadn't realized at the time is that all of their systems cut glucose load by using selected principles from the ones discussed above. Here's how:

- Dr. Atkins drops glucose load remarkably by cutting out nearly all carbohydrates from his diet.
- Dr. Barry Sears in *The Zone* uses three principles: He drops the carbohydrate in the diet from 60 to 40 percent and increases protein to 30 percent and fat to 30 percent.
- Dr. Ornish drops carbohydrate load by prescribing unrefined carbohydrates. It may appear to be a subtle point, but these carbos have a lower glycemic index so the glucose load is lowered, and it isn't possible to eat as many carbos if they're not refined, so the total amount of carbohydrate is reduced.
- Overeaters Anonymous. Their prescription for weight loss couldn't be simpler or more effective. Their slogan is: "No fat, no flour, no sugar." That means they eat none of the following:

cake	sugar
candy	sugared soft drinks
candy-coated gum	syrups
catsup	creamed, fried, or scalloped foods
cookies	refined cereals
honey	noodles and spaghetti
jam	beer, wine, alcoholic beverages
jelly	condensed milk
nuts	cream cheese
pastries	sour cream or whipped cream
peanut butter	crackers
pie	all bread products

Janice Kirata, who lost fifty-five pounds in four months, told me what it did for her. "When I put down the sugar, I wasn't so crazy anymore. I was a raging mother; now I'm calm. I'm more patient and not so stressed. I feel that it has given me a peace of mind and clarity that I didn't realize I was missing. When you're into the flour and sugar, your mind doesn't work right. When you get off it, you go through withdrawal. It's cleansing. Some people get tired or get headaches, but you come out of that and feel great. People lose the weight and keep it off."

All four diets cut glucose load and may well work for you to lose weight. The major consideration becomes which diet is healthiest in the long term. The answer is determined by what the diet does to your blood cholesterol and triglyceride levels as measured in your doctor's office. You should review these diets, if you are considering them, with your doctor for any risks or benefits they may pose. I chose Dean Ornish's diet for my mother because she needed to lower her cholesterol level, which the diet did.

HOW TO LOWER YOUR INSULIN LEVEL

First you need to know if your insulin level is elevated. The next time you have blood work, ask your doctor to include an insulin level test. It's available at most commercial labs. The insulin level is measured after an overnight fast. A lean person's fasting insulin measures out at 79, where that of an obese individual runs up to 190. You can imagine what a difference that much more insulin can make in producing and storing fat. If you can't measure your insulin level, here's a simple test you can perform yourself. Pinch a roll of fat next to your bellybutton; if you find more than an inch and a quarter, there's too much, according to Dr. Scott Grundy of the University of Texas in Dallas. (See the Appendix for the pinching technique.) That much fat directly under the skin around your naval predicts a high insulin level.

If your insulin level is elevated, the first step is to decrease your glucose load following the steps outlined above. That's likely to make a very large dent. There are a variety of supplements such as chromium and vanadyl sulfate, drugs, minerals, meal plans, and exercise programs that can help you further lower your insulin level to lose weight. They are fully outlined in the Appendix.

part two   *The Arsenal: Foods That Make You Lean*

Hard Foods, Hard Bodies

FOODS THAT MAKE YOU THIN

Stand in front of the mirror. Now open your mouth. What do you
see? With a full set of teeth there should be twenty plant crushers and
twelve flesh-ripping incisors. Pretty nice equipment, but for what?
Ice cream? Croissants? French fries? Swill? Not according to the design specifications. Yet you could eat most modern foods with no
teeth at all, a solid set of gums performing nicely. Your teeth were designed for tearing apart real foods . . . hard foods . . . and grinding
them into a coarse pulp, because those are the foods Mother Nature
intended us to eat. Your back teeth are a set of supercharged mortars
and pestles, which grind and break down great plant-based foods to
unlock disease-fighting phytochemicals, slow-release factors, fibers,
minerals, and vitamins. The front incisors and canines are meant to
tear apart tough, game meat, not melt-in-your-mouth hamburger
and pasta. John Heinerman, Ph.D., a medical anthropologist, says:
"The teeth and jaws of our cave man predecessors were a lot stronger
and more massive." Because cooked and refined foods required less
chewing, the size of molars, grinders, and jaw structure actually decreased. Over the course of several thousand years, the individuals
that evolved, that's us, are more gracile — effeminate . . . males included. Talk about going soft! What a bunch of sissies we've turned
into! These changes weren't from genetic mutations or natural selection. They were the results of a "use it or lose it" phenomenon, and
we've lost it. Now look at our intestines. They're thirty feet long. The
purpose of the whole rig is to digest hard foods. With modern soft
foods, we could get by with the first six inches because the foods are

completely digested by the time they would have reached inch number seven. But look at hard foods. Even when they're swallowed, they resist digestion. Parts of them are never digested at all. All hard foods give your entire intestine a really good workout, burning far more calories than slop and even increasing your metabolic rate. Hard foods, like hard woods, are slow-release superfuels that feed the body just the right amount of fuel it needs for a smooth quiet ride.

Conventional Wisdom
Soft foods, big belly.

LEAN
Hard foods, hard body.

ROAD MAP

This chapter rates carbohydrates and fats and proteins for their "hardness" factors or resistance to digestion. For each of these three groups there are truly hard foods, soft foods, and faux hard foods (foods that appear to be hard but are not). Throughout all the sections in this chapter, you will find charts that list those foods with the best hardness and weight-loss properties: low glucose load, high-soluble fiber, and high bulk. Eat these hard foods, and you will be lean. Soft foods and faux hard foods will make you fat. The special prominence of proteins earns them their very own chapter, which follows this one.

FOODS THAT MAKE YOU LEAN

Eat hard foods, and you cannot be fat, no matter how much you try to eat. Hard foods act as a natural brake against weight gain. They kill your appetite and keep your insulin at rock bottom. The more hard foods you eat, the leaner you will be. After he parked his F-16 nose-down in Bosnia, Captain Scott O'Grady survived on hard foods, namely bugs. Hard foods by their nature will dramatically cut your hunger and shut down the fat hormone insulin. A selection of the right ones will make your brain feel great.

My friend Charles Gaines, a body builder and author of *Pumping Iron,* who fortuitously wrote the book *Staying Hard,* has always believed in hard foods. Look at him and you can tell that's what he was bred on. He has a muscular leanness at fifty that most would-be hard bodies would kill for at twenty. He is a latter-day hunter-gatherer, eating lean game meats and vegetables. I introduced him to the carbo-loading phase at its peak. He rejected carbos and remained lean on hard foods with an exercise program that was modest in duration, al-though of a great intensity. I embraced stacks of carbos and needed ninety minutes of cycling, skating, running, or cross-country skiing in hopes of remaining lean.

Here's a look at the hard foods that will make you trim and keep you trim . . . and the soft foods that spell disaster.

CARBOHYDRATES
AMERICA GOES MARBLES

When Entenmann's came out with their low-fat coffee cake I took one taste and said, "Wow. This is really low in fat. It's all complex car-bohydrates. It must be really good for you. It tastes awesome. I bet I could eat the whole thing." And then I did. The biggest nutritional fraud ever hoisted on the American public was the idea that starches are health foods. Who could ever believe that the starchy foods everyone thought made you fat, everyone *knew* made you fat in the 1950s suddenly became the stay-thin health foods. What a joke! Huge hulking men trying to make themselves thin on pizza! Fashion mod-els trying to remain employable on big bowls of pasta. But it was a great high concept: to enjoy the very core of recreational eating while you lose weight. Starches are largely responsible for the fatten-ing of America. Think about it. When stockyards fatten cattle for prime grade beef, they don't give them sour cream and butter, they give them starches, masses of them. Starches do the same for people, marbling them until the fat appears to pop through the skin. If you have any doubts, remember that we eat a smaller percent of fat in our diet now than ten years ago, but have gained an average of eight pounds during the same period. In the 1980s, the peak of the health boom, men aged thirty to thirty-nine gained four pounds, while women gained nine pounds. Our kids are the fattest they've ever been! Those seriously overweight jumped 30 percent in the same decade. Who's to blame? Starches, lots of them, many under the guise of "low-fat foods" that, while low in fat, are packed with highly fattening refined carbos. Most people realize that the simple carbohydrates found in candies can make you fat. But what they don't realize is that loads of starches can make you a great deal fatter.

Conventional Wisdom
Starches are health foods.

LEAN
Starches fuel massive weight gain.

HARD CARBOHYDRATES

These are the hearty fuels the human body was designed for. Quite simply, these are complex carbos that take a very long time to enter your bloodstream after you eat them. Your teeth have to rip, grind, and chew them vigorously. The enzymes in your stomach have to fight to pull them apart because the starches are covered by a hardened case. They have lots of fiber to slow their absorption and blunt their effect on blood sugar and cholesterol. By leaving carbos in the packaging that nature provides, they remain tremendously healthful foods.

Look for these five key characteristics, all of which give hard carbos a slow release of sugars into the blood and a low-insulin response:

- Low GI: Hard foods barely bump your blood sugar or insulin at all. They are found at the bottom of the glycemic index scale. Look for a complete listing of low-GI foods in the chapter "Hard Beans."
- High fiber: Fibers make hard foods hard. Look for lots of fiber, a minimum of 5 grams printed on the label of processed foods. Great Northern beans have 9 grams per serving. The chapter "Hard Fibers" has a complete listing of foods that have hard fiber.
- Still hard when ready to eat: After final food preparations are made, hard foods are still firm to hard to the touch and to the bite.
- Physically large: Hard carbos have a large physical size like bulgur cracked wheat with its big, chunky cracked segments of the grain. They are coarse, not fine to the touch.
- Robust sugars: Doongara rice has a glycemic index of 66. Parboiled rice has a GI of 93. The difference is that the Doongara rice is very

high in a sugar called amylose. Bret Goodpaster, Ph.D., found that amylose was digested more incompletely than the sugars amylopectin or glucose, making it far more robust. "This is because of its chemical structure. It's digested less and more incompletely. It's not as bioavailable. The sugars in them are nondigestible."

WRECKED HARD CARBOS

Many carbos that are hard in their natural state are ruined in processing or cooking. Just as you can wilt a perfectly good piece of broccoli into a limp dishrag, you can pound, steam, or boil the hardest beans into slop. Now they're still better than really soft carbos because they've got some fiber in them, but the more you soften, refine, and grind up food, the less work your own teeth and digestive enzymes have to do. The less work they have to do, the quicker sugars enter into your system and the fatter you'll be. Refined, overcooked, milled carbos of all shapes and forms can blast your blood sugar and insulin into low earth orbit.

SMALL SIZE

Ethnobotanist Gary Nabhan says, "In general, the smaller the particle size, the more rapidly absorbed the sugar is from any food. Take oatmeal, for instance. When it is ground down to a powder — as it is in Mueslix cereals — that powdery dust has a quicker absorption time and is more easily dissolved into a sugary mush." Muesli has a GI well into the high category. Grinding carbos down to a smaller particle size creates a greater surface area, so digestive enzymes have more to work on and can speed digestion. Grinding grains into a fine powder is going to give you the greatest surface area. The finer the food, the quicker it is digested. Ground rice, for example, digests much faster than whole rice.

HEAT

Starch comes in sacs, some of which are pretty formidable and resist digestion until they are ruptured. Heat and water cause the starch to swell and to change its physical properties, so it becomes more like a simple sugar. This process, called gelatinization, allows the enzymes in the stomach and small intestine to attack the starch and dissolve it. Chuck Weber, a professor in the department of nutritional sciences at the University of Arizona, College of Agriculture, says, "If you eat raw potato starch, you'll get a digestibility of about 30 percent. If you heat treat it, you'll get a digestibility of about 90 percent. The starch itself will become exposed to the enzyme amylase much more quickly after it's wetted and heated." Dehydrated beans have become very popular. "Just add boiling water," say the directions. But you will find many of these dishes become mush. Take ordinary white rice. Boiling it for fifteen minutes instead of five minutes increases the GI by 150 percent.

In short, blood sugar levels and insulin responses depend on particle size and cooking time as well as the type of cooking process. Previous studies showed lower responses to home-cooked food compared with their processed equivalents. Experts believe that the traditional methods used in the preparation of meals is what contributed to their slow-release nature.

FAUX HARD CARBOS

Hard carbos are naturally hard, yet you can buy a wide variety of carbohydrates that will give your teeth a good crunchy sound when you chew. There's little disputing that they are hard, but they are not naturally so. Take a crunchy breakfast cereal. I remember an oat bran cereal that was my favorite until I read the new nutritional labels. Sure, it had lots of oats, but it was packed with 22 grams of sugar. What makes the oats hard? Transfatty acids. These have been around since the original Crisco in 1911. They are fats that make everything from potato chips to breakfast cereals crunchy and hard. This fat may be the worst of all for your heart, not to mention what it does to your waistline. Transfatty acids are the primary hardening ingredient used in processed foods. Although the oats in this cereal might have put it low on the glycemic index category, the masses of sugars in the preparation raise its glycemic index considerably. A more classic faux hard food is a potato chip. This is a high glycemic index food that is peeled, fried, and fat-hardened.

Food manufacturers switched to much safer sounding vegetable oils when forced by public opinion to give up the saturated fats in processed foods. However, to impart the same qualities that were loved in saturated fats, the manufacturers created a risk of heart disease, gram for gram, up to three times higher, according to Harvard's Dr. Walter Willett. Those qualities are hardness at room temperature for easy storage and adding crispness and texture to foods. You can tell these foods by the words "hydrogenated" or "partially hydrogenated" oils on their labels. These are the "hidden" fats that we usually don't count in our diet, preferring to believe that they are healthful vegetable oils. Examples include:

- Hard margarine
- Cookies
- Cakes
- Potato chips
- Many bakery items
- Tortillas
- Many packaged convenience foods

SOFT CARBOHYDRATES

Have you ever read diet books that encourage you to chew your food? With hard foods, those instructions are silly — you have no choice. With soft carbos, why bother? Soft carbos don't take any chewing at all. Your body wants to offer some defense against these fast-burning carbos, but the last line of defense has already been stripped away by milling machines and the other tools of the food-processing trade. Many of these foods dissolve quickly in your mouth. Unfortunately, they'll do the same in your intestine . . . literally dissolving into your bloodstream with little resistance. That's because many complex carbos are just big packages of glucose, which can drive your blood sugar level far higher and far faster than table sugar. As an example, a piece of white bread speeds glucose into your system 40 percent faster than sugar! Eating soft carbos, in the belief that they are health foods, is the biggest single food error that weight-conscious Americans continue to make. Soft carbos are the number-one food that Americans eat, according to the National Center for Health Statistics. When we dump all that extra sugar into our system we're saying, "Make me fat!" If we add fat to it, it's like saying, "Make me look like Santa." Soft carbos are digested in the first foot of intestine and shoot carbos into the bloodstream far faster than they can be used, like a carburetor spilling fuel into an engine. Even if you were running at a marathon pace, your body couldn't use glucose as fast as soft carbos throw them at your system.

Soft carbos never have a chance from the get-go. Each one of these characteristics ensures soft carbos a fast ride through your digestive system, with a sharp rise in blood sugar and an outright hostile insulin response.

- High GI: rank higher than sugar on the glycemic index scale
- Weak sugars: easy to digest carbohydrate molecules
- Low fiber
- Soft after cooking
- Physically small and refined particles (these have a much larger surface area for digestive enzymes to work on)

The easiest way to remember soft carbos is that they're just that . . . soft. You barely need to chew at all. Here are some examples:

- White rice
- Pancakes
- Coffee cake
- Pasta
- White bread

STEALTH FOODS

These are foods that evade your body's ability to protect itself from them, which they do in two key ways. First, they evade any natural satiety mechanism. You won't feel satisfied until you've eaten far too much. Second, they are quickly absorbed into the body. Your body can't put up any resistance. All flour foods, high-fat foods, ice creams, sugary frozen yogurts are examples of stealth foods. You *can* eat stealth foods, but only if you've preloaded your system with foods that are already working hard on your satiety centers and that can slow the absorption of food from your gut. It is quite true that once food moves down in your intestine it is one big broth into which all the different foods you have eaten are contained, but the more hard foods and fibers you have, the more resistant you are to effects of stealth foods.

There are two ingredients in particular that lead the list of stealth food ingredients you need to watch for.

CORN SYRUP

We each eat 51.7 pounds of high-fructose corn syrup a year reports the Department of Agriculture's *Economic Research Service Report,* an increase of 25 pounds from the mid-1980s. However, most of us make no conscious effort to eat corn syrup. The consumption has risen because corn syrup is now used in everything from soft drinks and tomato sauce to breads, crackers, and cereals. Most of the "sugar" we eat is corn syrup. Corn syrup is much cheaper than sugar, honey, or molasses, costing $4 a pound less than Midwest beet sugar.

WHITE FLOUR

Eating pure white flour products is worse than mainlining sugar. "The body handles white flour like sugar by digesting it very quickly," says nutritional scientist Dr. Luke Bucci. Dr. Judith Hall-frisch of the USDA says, "White flour is very efficiently absorbed. White bread is used as the base for the glycemic index by Jenkins. So really it's not much different from glucose."

When whole wheat is milled into white flour, as much as 83 percent of the nutrients are removed, with mostly starch remaining. The fiber is gone, and the vitamin E content is reduced, along with twenty-one other nutrients, so it must be fortified with synthetically manufactured thiamin, riboflavin, niacin, and iron. White flour is also adulterated with chemicals used to age, whiten, and preserve the product. White flour is found in many of the foods considered healthiest, such as bagels, pastas, breads, and cereals. If you are having trouble losing unwanted fat, consider dropping white flour products first. Beware of products that say "wheat flour," which usually indicates highly processed flour with caramel coloring. If it says "whole wheat," the FDA stipulates that it must be whole wheat.

FRUIT

Even though it won't drive up your blood sugar level, the sugar in fruit will make you plenty fat. Fructose goes to the liver as a sugar, but returns to the bloodstream as a fat called a triglyceride. Hard fruits, like Macintosh apples, are low in fructose and high in slow-release factors called pectins. They are listed in the chapter "Hard Fruits." Soft fruits like bananas are high in fructose and have minimal slow-release capabilities. Bananas also have a high glycemic index. If you are giving up sugary snacks and foods, beware of overdosing on fruit. In an effort to get the same endorphin high that sugars deliver, you may overeat fruit hoping to get that same high, but you won't because fructose has no effect on brain endorphins.

ALCOHOL CARBOS

Canadian researchers demonstrated that men and women consuming alcohol with their meals increased their caloric intake far beyond what they really needed, particularly if they ate fatty foods. Most of us made that observation the first time we ate a whole large pizza in college after downing a six-pack of beer. If protein is the food that satiates fastest, alcohol is the food that satiates least. Dr. Angelo Tremblay, a professor of nutrition and physiology at Laval University in Ste.-Foy, Quebec, concluded that the brain just doesn't register the calories that the body's taken in from alcoholic beverages, so your body won't compensate by ingesting fewer calories. Excess energy taken in as either alcohol or fat promotes fat storage. Worse still, alcohol suppresses the breakdown of fat, which makes alcohol and fat a potent formula for accelerated weight gain. And that's all with a single 12-ounce glass of 7 percent beer!

THE FRENCH PARADOX

A yacht designer took me aside last summer in St.-Tropez. He said, "You Americans eat junk food and become horribly fat. We French eat like pigs and we are not so fat." The French are widely envied for their spectacular food and even more so for their ability to eat it without becoming morbidly obese. In fact, judged by the average French figure on the Côte d'Azur, they look pretty trim. Most Americans want to know how they can stay so thin and eat so much fat. The answer is simple: The French are operating with one hand tied behind the back — they eat few soft carbos. The *Wall Street Journal* reports that the sale of baguettes, one of the fastest-burning carbos of all, has dropped precipitously in France precisely because the French fear that baguettes will make them fat. The French simply lack the nutritional machinery to make themselves fat. The French even have a foie grâs diet. The inventor of that diet, Michel Montignac, agrees that the low-fat, low-calorie diet was one of the great swindles of the century. His diet restricts soft carbos from starches and sweets to alcohol. Skeptics worry about its huge amounts of fat, but the program does prove the point: Soft carbos make you fat, and dumping them makes you thinner. His cult diet books encourage the consumption of great-tasting foods. But if you look closely, you'll see that his duck and sausage stew is stocked with hard carbos in the form of white beans. In a word, the French have the most elegant way on earth to cut the glucose load: they drop refined flours and add incredibly great-tasting fats. The French also win by eating most of their calories at lunch, which increases their metabolism during the afternoon and evening. Their regular consumption of wines makes the fat less dangerous to the heart, but gives them seven times the death rate of cirrhosis of the liver found in the U.S. Now a word of warning. This is in no way to suggest that you adapt a high-saturated-fat diet to lose weight or to become healthy. The French paradox simply drives home the point that soft carbos are the number-one villain when it comes to making people fat.

FATS

An active imagination isn't required to figure out that fats are the softest of soft foods. Butter, vegetable oils, shortening, bacon, French fries, and ice cream make real body fat with alarming speed, no matter what anyone claims. The body doesn't demand any special effort to store fat as fat. Where turning fat into sugar at least takes some effort, fat is locked, loaded, and aimed at your belly and thighs as soon as it enters your stomach. Dr. James Stubbs of the Rowett Institute says, "Fatter people consume a higher proportion of their energy intake from fat than from carbohydrate." The more fat you eat, the fatter you'll be. Mixed with fast-burning "soft" carbos and a high insulin level, fats move into fat cells with the speed of a bullet train. We widely assume that fat is passé as a cause of being fat. The assumption is that we've all cut our fat by such a degree that we're now fat virgins, where the stuff never crosses our lips. Wrong. The HANES III government survey confirms that Americans eat more grams of fat than ever before, although the percentage of fat we eat has decreased. Here's where the math comes in. While we've increased the amount of fat we eat, we've increased the number of carbos even more. That obscures the increase in fat by diluting it with all those extra carbohydrate calories. More simply put, we eat so many more junk carbos that we've obscured the fact that we're eating more fat too. More fat and more soft carbos produce a one plus one equals ten equation. Neither alone would make us as fat as the combination.

Conventional Wisdom

Fat in moderation.

LEAN

No fat, no fat.

HARD FATS

The word "fat" is the popular terminology for a fatty acid. It's the fatty acids that are actually found in foods, transported in the blood, and locked into fat cells. The category "hard fats" is a term for hard foods that contain fatty acids. The following fats have potential health benefits as long as they are part of foods and not taken as supplements. These are the only fats you'll want to ingest. First among them are the essential fatty acids — arachidonic, linoleic, and linolenic acids (found in olive oil, canola oil, flaxseed oil, soybean, salmon, and sunflower seed oil, as well as seeds, nuts, and green vegetables)— required to make good prostaglandins that make sertonin work better. One radical theory holds that a shortage of them may cause coronary artery disease. Second are the Omega 3 fatty acids found in fish, which may play a role in heart disease and stroke prevention. Third are the monounsaturated fats that lower bad cholesterol levels without lowering the good cholesterol.

FAUX FAT

The latest, hottest food triumph from nutritional engineers is the artificial fat Olestra. This gives products the look, feel, and texture of fat but adds no fat or calories at all. After nearly three decades of research and $200 million in development, you are subtracting 90 calories of fat from a bag of potato chips. No mean feat. But on the minus side of the balance sheet, you are taking nutrients called carotenoids out of other foods that are in your digestive tract at the same time. So, for instance, if you ate a sweet potato, a cantaloupe, and a carrot, the Olestra would prevent those foods' most valuable nutrients, the carotenoids, from being absorbed into your body. Since these are extremely powerful cancer and heart disease fighting substances, Dr. Walter Willett of the Harvard School of Public Health fears that this could lead to a rash of new cancers twenty years from now. The FDA has approved Olestra in these savory snacks: potato chips, cheese curls, cheese puffs, cookies, crackers, and tortilla chips. Dr. Willett worries that many of the healthful chips presently on the market containing canola oil, which is known to lower cholesterol levels, will have the canola oil replaced with Olestra by the manufacturer, removing the only healthful part of the food. That brings up the other point. The advent of these products may cause dieters to binge, believing that these low-fat foods will help them stay thin. But since they are made almost entirely of fast-burning carbos, they will have the unintended effect of raising blood insulin, cholesterol, triglycerides, and blood sugar levels. Now if Olestra were added to superhealthful hard carbos and led more people to eat them, I think they'd have an argument, especially if you were certain to eat your carotenoid-rich foods at other times of the day when Olestra wouldn't interfere. However, those products have not yet appeared. On a more practical level, if you are going to eat an Olestra product, don't eat it with your beta-carotenoid-rich fruits and vegetables such as sweet potato, carrot, and cantaloupe. Because Olestra takes carotenoids from foods that are in the gut at the same time it is, Olestra is of potential harm only when those carotenoid-rich foods are in the digestive tract at the same time. Olestra is also a terrific way to push up glucose load, by creating a product with fast-burning high-GI carbos, little fiber, and no fat to cut glucose load. Dr. Willett worries that this will sharply increase the glucose load of the diet. A newer product, originally designed for people with diabetes to control their blood sugar, is called Z-trim. It's actually made from the fibrous outer coating of grains and could prove to be quite healthy.

SOFT FATS

The softest soft fats are oils, which are the densest concentration of calories on earth. No matter how healthful someone may proclaim that a vegetable oil is or how good gravy may taste, these are the foods that make you fattest. Examples include:
- Vegetable oils
- Gravy
- Butter
- Whole milk: An eight-ounce serving of whole milk has eight grams of fat. Eight ounces of 1 percent milk still contains two to three grams of fat.

KINDS OF FATS

LONG-CHAIN SATURATED FATS

These will send your cholesterol level flying higher than any other food. They're the most dangerous food ingredient that isn't labeled with a skull and crossbones. The government says you can eat 10 percent of your calories as saturated fats. *Consumer Reports* recommends 7 percent. In truth, you don't need any. Examples include fats found in:
- Red meat
- Butter
- Eggs
- Cheese
- Coconut and palm oils

SHORT-CHAIN FATTY ACIDS

These are manufactured in your large colon from fiber in your food. They may have great health benefits, from the protection against colon cancer to lowering your blood cholesterol. You don't actually eat these. They are manufactured from fiber in your colon.   ★★★★

MONOUNSATURATED FATS

These have been the glory fats for the last several years. Studies show they lower your bad cholesterol without lowering your good cholesterol. This is the core concept behind the Mediterranean diet's high admissible fat content and the reason that olive oil has been so widely promoted. The prestigious Dallas Southwestern Medical Center team doesn't believe they have much advantage over polyunsaturated fats if taken in small to moderate amounts. However, if you eat most of your fat calories as olive oil, as people in some Mediterranean countries do, then monounsaturated fats will put your blood cholesterol on much more favorable terms. Examples include:
- Olive oil
- Canola oil, a close substitute for olive oil   *****

POLYUNSATURATED FATS

These were long sold as safer than saturated fats. Unadulterated polyunsaturated fats such as pure vegetable oils have, in studies, been shown to lower bad cholesterol levels but have the misfortune of also lowering good cholesterol levels. Examples include:
- Corn oil
- Liquid margarine

PROTEINS

In their purest state, proteins are the foods most immediately satisfying to the appetite. Because of their renewed prominence in many modern diets, the entire next chapter is devoted to proteins.

Hard foods resist the body's effort to quickly digest them because they are physically harder to chew, and slower to break down. That means that blood sugar doesn't rise quickly, insulin stays low, and sugar doesn't turn to fat. These slow-burning foods prevent the blood sugar crashes that cause intense hunger and make your brain feel bad. Since hard foods are bulkier and fill you up fuller and quicker, you can't overeat.

BE TOUGH TO EAT HARD

Look at someone who's lean. The first word that comes to mind in describing that person is "tough," like my brother Doug. He was always leaner, more agile, and tougher than I was. He became captain of his college football team, then ran World Cup Soccer and even became chief of the Olympic Games in Atlanta. He ate hard foods growing up, I ate soft foods. I'm convinced that's why he's tougher across the board. Now, you'd think that people like my brother exert enormous amounts of effort to stay as lean as they do. Curiously, they may do less exercise than you and put in far less overall effort to control their food intake. That difference certainly exists between my brother and me. He's tough, however, where it really counts, pushing away the wrong foods at the dinner table. Tough men and women choose hard foods. It may sound silly that you have to be tough when you eat, but most of us do gravitate to soft foods. We're like junkies looking for the quick druglike hit. OK, we're convinced: Hard foods are a great idea. But who the hell can eat the stuff? Just remember that quick hits of any kind are short lived and need to be countered with additional foods. Be tough enough to wait for hard foods to deliver their long-lasting punch, tremendous depth of strength, inner peace, and leanness, and you will become mentally tough about the foods that you eat. The biggest part of being mentally tough is making your brain feel good. Hard foods go down harder than soft foods. They take a lot more effort to select, chew, and digest, but the end effect on satiety and brain function is remarkable. They feel great, so you can look great. So be tough! Eat the hard foods that make you hard! Food selection is easy. You will find that you simply cannot remain fat if you eat only hard foods.

Just exactly how tough can eating be? It's not like swinging a sledgehammer on a rockpile or working on a double shift at an automotive plant. It's just eating.

Protein

Protein has earned a decades-long reputation as the most commercially successful food group for dieters. From the legendary Dr. Atkins and the liquid protein diets of the 1970s to books such as *The Zone* and *Protein Power,* many of the most successful diet books have hung their hats on protein.

Conventional Wisdom
Americans eat too much protein.

LEAN
Protein power keeps you lean.

ROAD MAP
You'll find all the answers to the more protein, less protein dilemma with an exacting system to determine just how much protein you really need. The chapter lists the hardest, hard-core proteins and the very best proteins for weight loss judged by having the least excess caloric baggage.

BENEFITS
Protein has three enormous weight-loss benefits.
- Satiating: Protein is a far superior hunger killer than either carbohydrate or fat.
- Brain energizing: Protein is the primary source of the amino acid tyrosine, which increases the production of the energizing neurotransmitters norepinephrine and dopamine.

- Insulin lowering: Protein decreases insulin production by signaling the pancreas to make glucagon.
- A carbo substitute: Protein serves as a carbo substitute, which decreases glucose load and therefore insulin.

PROTEIN CONFUSION

There is a great deal of confusion about just how much protein you should eat. Old school nutritionists insist that we all eat far too much and need never even consider protein when we eat. The latest diets suggest nearly tripling the percent of protein in your diet, from 12 to 30 percent. I favor 20 to 25 percent during the period you are shedding fat. We'll look at the safety issues at the end of this chapter.

HOW TO DETERMINE YOUR PROTEIN NEEDS

Like many pasta-stuffing aerobic junkies, many of my friends and I ignored protein for years. We found ourselves weak and hobbled after workouts, overtrained and overtired. The mistake we made was eating too little quality protein. Dieters often eat so little quality protein that they destroy their own muscle to get enough for the body's needs. Here's a simple way of determining how much protein you need based on your activity level and how to use it strategically in your diet to control your weight.

Step one: Determine your level of physical activity.

Level 1: You are sedentary, do light weight training or less than 40 minutes of aerobics a day.
Level 2: You are a seasoned body builder who trains four days a week.
Level 3: You are a serious aerobic athlete training 60–90 minutes a day.
Level 4: You are just beginning a program of building substantial amounts of muscle and plan to train at least four days a week.
Level 5: You are a professional athlete.

Step two: Determine how many grams of protein you require in a day. First, find your activity level along the top of the next table. Fol-

Maximum Grams of Protein Intake per Day

Weight	Level of Activity				
(in pounds)	1	2	3	4	5
100	36g	55g	59g	77g	91g
110	40	60	65	85	100
120	44	65	71	93	109
130	47	71	77	100	118
140	51	76	83	108	127
150	55	82	89	116	136
160	58	87	95	124	145
170	62	93	100	131	155
180	65	98	106	139	164
190	69	104	112	147	173
200	73	109	118	155	182
210	76	115	124	162	191
220	80	120	130	170	200
230	84	125	136	178	209
240	87	131	142	185	218
250	91	136	148	193	227
260	95	142	154	201	236

low down that column until you find the number opposite your weight in pounds. That's the maximum grams of protein intake per day for which there is at least some scientific evidence of efficacy.

If you are concerned about safety, have your doctor draw a test for blood urea nitrogen to ascertain if you are overloading. If this sounds dangerous, keep in mind that the average American on a red meat and potatoes diet eats the amount of protein suggested for Level 4. On days you don't train, you don't need the extra protein. Remember that clean proteins that come from vegetable sources and are low in fat don't lead to diabetes, hypertension, or heart disease; in fact, they may prevent them.

Step three: Learn how to use protein strategically. Plan meals around your protein intake, then add quality, hard carbohydrates. Eat protein as your first food of the day to get your brain feeling great. Right after exercise is the next best opportunity, since protein can supply new muscle at that time. Eat protein with midmorning and midafternoon snacks as well as lunch to stay sharp. Carbohydrate meals without protein make most men drowsy, while women find them calming. Since too much protein in the evening makes it hard to fall asleep, I eat less protein and more carbos for a late evening snack. By including protein in all your meals and snacks as a satiator, you'll cut down on the amount you eat. I've always eaten a big breakfast, at least 700 calories. I was still ravenously hungry by noon and could pack away another 1,000 calories. By increasing my morning protein, I almost have to force myself to eat lunch. Here's a summary of how to use protein.

- Eat at the beginning of each meal to satiate your hunger in order to prevent overeating.
- Include adequate amounts in all daytime meals and snacks to prevent overeating.
- Use higher concentrations in the morning and early afternoon to make your workday more productive.
- Use a protein supplement in your sports drink to increase endurance, concentration, and psyche.
- Use in the evening only if you have to be sharp and alert.

Take the total amount of protein you're going to eat for a day. Say that's 100 grams. Use 25 to start your day with breakfast, 15 for your midmorning snack, 25 for lunch, 15 for your midafternoon snack. Then 10 for dinner and 10 for your late-night snack. Take as much as you can in a protein food such as a glass of milk, piece of fish, or bowl of soybeans so that you get its most concentrated effect. This seems like a simple point, but most of us get a big dose of protein diluted within other foods so we never get the concentrated satiating and energizing effects of nearly pure protein. Rather than tripling your protein intake, make the maximum of what you do eat so you enjoy its effects by eating it or drinking it straight up.

Since there is no storage form of protein, you can use only so much at a sitting. Experts put that at about 30 grams.

Step Four: Eat hard proteins. Hard proteins are exceptionally low in fats and carbohydrates. They are tough to chew and digest. Soft proteins, high fats, sugar, and calcium pose the real dangers of proteins. What follows are hard-core proteins.

HARD PROTEINS

HARD BEANS

Hard beans are firm and take real grinding to dissolve into little pieces. They cut your appetite and lower your insulin. They are the most healthful foods discussed in this book, which is why there is an entire chapter on them.

HARD DAIRY

Americans think of red meats as the most choice protein, when in fact dairy proteins are rated number one for muscle-building protein quality. Lean dairy products are great satiators, quite convenient and good energizers. Since there's no need to rip and tear and digestion proceeds quickly, they aren't strictly "hard" proteins. However, the faster digestion time can be used to your advantage to deliver the satiating and energizing power of protein more quickly. Hard dairy products are those that haven't been adulterated with fats. They include skim milk, low-fat yogurt without added sugar, egg whites, whey protein, and low-fat cottage cheese.

OTHER LEAN PROTEINS

The table below lists proteins from hard to squishy. The rating system ranks the protein from the least number of excess or nonprotein calories to the greatest. Nonprotein or "excess" calories refers to the total number of fat and carbohydrate calories. For instance, egg whites have no wasted calories at all whereas low-fat fruit-flavored yogurt has a total of 192 out of 227 calories that are not protein. You could better have used those calories to have a plate of vegetables or bowl of beans. These kinds of foods make protein extremely "expensive" to eat in terms of extra calories.

Since most proteins have little fiber, there is no built-in protection against the extra carbos and fat. So use those proteins near the top of the list for the leanest bang. One exception: Fish may appear to score poorly because of the higher fat content. However, remember that the Omega 3 fatty acids actually help to lower insulin levels by changing the muscle membrane so that less insulin is required.

Lean Proteins

Product	Amount	Calories	Protein (grams)	Fat (grams)	Total Carbos	Excess Nonprotein Calories
Nonfat vanilla yogurt	1 cup	195	12	0	0	0
Protein powder, soy	2 heaping Tbsp	80	18	0	0	0
Protein powder, egg	2 heaping Tbsp	100	24	0	0	0
Egg white	1 large	16	3.4	0	0.6	2
Greenland turbot	3 oz.	74	14.7	0.3		3
Protein powder, milk	2 heaping Tbsp	110	25	0	1	4
Snow Crab	3 oz.	84	18.3	0.6		5
Croaker	3 oz.	82	17.9	0.63		6
Lingcod	3 oz.	87	19	0.64		6
Pacific cod	3 oz.	82	17.8	0.67		6
Dolphin	3 oz.	87	19	0.69		6
Walleye pike	3 oz.	88	19.3	0.69		6
Cod, baked	3 oz.	89	19.4	0.7	0	6
Eel	3 oz.	85	18.5	0.7		6
Snapper	3 oz.	89	19.6	0.7		6
Halibut	3 oz.	87	18.9	0.72		6
Clams (raw)	3 oz.	105	17.1	0.76		7
Shrimp	3 oz.	88	16.8	0.76		7
Pompano	3 oz.	81	17.2	0.8		7
Carp	3 oz.	90	19.3	0.81		7
Atlantic herring	3 oz.	102	21.9	0.9		8
Spiny lobster	3 oz.	90	18.8	0.9		8
Whitefish	3 oz.	108	23.4	0.95		9
Mahimahi (dolphin fillet)	3 oz.	108	23.4	0.95		9
Blue crab	3 oz.	74	12.8	0.97		9
King crab	3 oz.	86	17.4	0.97		9
Alaskan pollock	3 oz.	92	19.4	0.98		9
Yellowfin tuna	3 oz.	103	22	1.01		9
Haddock	3 oz.	92	19.4	1.02		9
Atlantic mackerel	3 oz.	85	17.7	1.06		10
Northern lobster	3 oz.	89	18.7	1.06		10
Dungeness crab	3 oz.	87	18.1	1.08		10
Hawaiian wahoo	3 oz.	94	19.3	1.1		10
Crayfish	3 oz.	90	18.5	1.18		11
Golden kingklip	3 oz.	91	18.8	1.19		11
Spot	3 oz.	91	18	1.19		11
Rainbow trout	3 oz.	93	19.1	1.22		11
Turbot	3 oz.	90	18.3	1.31		12

Lean Proteins (cont.)

Product	Amount	Calories	Protein (grams)	Fat (grams)	Total Carbos	Excess Nonprotein Calories
Sole	3 oz.	100	20.5	1.34		12
Orange roughy	3 oz.	91	18.5	1.4		13
Mussels (blue)	3 oz.	112	20.6	1.51		14
Mullet	3 oz.	76	14.5	1.52		14
Sablefish	3 oz.	94	18.8	1.57		14
Pacific ocean perch	3 oz.	94	18.6	1.63		15
Butterfish	3 oz.	98	20.7	1.7		15
Snails (unspec. raw)	3 oz.	106	20.3	1.73		16
Nonfat cottage cheese	1 cup	123	28	0.6	2.7	16
Cusk	3 oz.	94	18.8	1.9		17
Squid	3 oz.	75	14.4	1.9		17
Pacific jack mackerel	3 oz.	105	20.3	2		18
Sea trout	3 oz.	97	18.4	2		18
Tuna, white, canned in water	3 oz.	116	22.7	2.1	0	19
Eastern and Gulf oysters	3 oz.	86	11.9	2.24		20
Bigeye tuna	3 oz.	110	20.8	2.29		21
Scallops	3 oz.	81	9.45	2.3		21
Opakapaka	3 oz.	124	24.1	2.3		21
Albacore tuna	3 oz.	96	17.5	2.31		21
Swordfish	3 oz.	97	17.7	2.33		21
Abalone	3 oz.	98	18.5	2.4		22
Tilapia	3 oz.	97	17.6	2.42		22
Pacific oysters	3 oz.	69	7.06	2.47		22
Atlantic cod	3 oz.	111	20.5	2.5		23
Whey protein — 80%	2 heaping Tbsp	100	20	1.8	2	24
Redfish	3 oz.	105	18.9	2.73		25
Chicken breast, no skin, roasted	3 oz.	142	26.7	3.1	0	28
Crevalle jack	3 oz.	104	17.8	3.17		29
Turkey breast, no skin, roasted	3.5 oz.	157	29.9	3.2	0	29
Shad, baked	3 oz.	118	20.6	3.36		30
Venison, lean, raw	3 oz.	107	17.9	3.4	0	31
Sockeye salmon	3 oz.	116	19.9	3.45		31
Grouper	3 oz.	99	16.9	3.5		32
Atlantic ocean perch	3 oz.	103	17.6	3.6		32
Shad	3 oz.	104	16.7	3.61		32
Ocean catfish	3 oz.	117	19.4	3.79		34

Lean Proteins (cont.)

Product	Amount	Calories	Protein (grams)	Fat (grams)	Total Carbos	Excess Nonprotein Calories
Tilefish	3 oz.	121	19.8	4.01		36
Blue runner	3 oz.	124	20	4.24		38
Lake trout	3 oz.	116	18.2	4.26		38
Skate (ray)	3 oz.	130	21	4.51		41
Pork tenderloin, trimmed, roasted	3.5 oz.	166	28.8	4.8	0	43
Rockfish	3 oz.	117	18.5	4.8		43
Bluefish	3 oz.	131	20.4	4.84		44
Reduced-fat cheese	1 oz.	73	6	4.5	0.8	44
Skipjack tuna	3 oz.	144	23.3	4.9		44
Striped bass	3 oz.	123	18.5	4.9		44
Yeast, dry baker's	1 oz.	80	10.5	0.5	11	49
Skim milk	1 cup	86	8	0.2	11.9	49
Catfish (channel)	3 oz.	127	17.8	5.6		50
Whiting	3 oz.	134	19.1	5.86		53
Egg, whole (chicken)	1 large	79	6.1	5.6	0.6	53
Pink salmon	3 oz.	146	21.6	5.95		54
Round steak, trimmed, broiled	3.5 oz.	191	31.7	6.2	0	56
Salmon, canned	3 oz.	130	17.4	6.2	0	56
Monkfish	3 oz.	139	19.3	6.3		57
Mozzarella cheese	1 oz.	80	7	6.1	0.6	57
Lake whitefish	3 oz.	148	20.8	6.61		59
Atlantic pollock	3 oz.	126	14.7	7		63
Northern pike	3 oz.	140	18.5	7.2		65
Buttermilk	1 cup	99	8	2.2	11.7	67
Bluefin tuna	3 oz.	177	25.3	7.6		68
Parmesan cheese	1 oz.	111	10	7.3	0.9	69
1% milk	1 cup	102	8	2.4	12.2	70
Provolone cheese	1 oz.	100	7	7.6	0.6	71
Spanish mackerel	3 oz.	157	20.1	7.89		71
Bonito	3 oz.	145	17.3	8.02		72
Cottage cheese, 2% fat	1 cup	203	31.1	4.4	8.2	72
Gouda cheese	1 oz.	101	7	7.8	0.6	73
Yogurt, plain nonfat	1 cup	140	14	0.4	17.4	73
Flounder, baked	3.5 oz.	202	30	8.2	0	74
Yogurt, nonfat frozen	½ cup	100	4	0.1	18.7	76
Atlantic sardines, canned, in oil	3 oz.	168	21.3	8.56		77
Monterey Jack cheese	1 oz.	106	8	8.6	0.2	78
Pacific herring	3 oz.	158	18	9.04		81

Lean Proteins (cont.)

Product	Amount	Calories	Protein (grams)	Fat (grams)	Total Carbos	Excess Nonprotein Calories
Porgy	3 oz.	164	18.5	9.47		85
Coho salmon	3 oz.	180	20.1	10.44		94
Yogurt, low-fat plain	1 cup	159	13	3.5	16	96
Pacific sardines, canned in tomato sauce	3 oz.	208	24.6	11.46		103
Flounder	3 oz.	184	18.4	11.66		105
Yogurt, low-fat frozen	½ cup	110	4	3.5	18.7	106
Sea bass	3 oz.	178	16.4	11.98		108
Part-skim ricotta cheese	½ cup	171	14	9.8	6.4	114
Smelt	3 oz.	197	16.9	13.77		124
Shark	3 oz.	197	16.9	13.77		124
Ling	3 oz.	195	16.4	13.88		125
King mackerel	3 oz.	205	18.6	13.89		125
Chocolate (1% fat) milk	1 cup	158	8	2.5	26.1	127
Chinook salmon	3 oz.	195	13.4	15.3		138
Ground beef, extra lean, baked	3.5 oz.	274	30.3	16	0	144
Yogurt, low-fat vanilla	1 cup	209	12	2.8	31.3	150
American cheese	2 oz. (slices)	212	12.6	17.8	1	164
Peanut butter, smooth	2 Tbsp	188	9	16	5.4	166
Yogurt, low-fat fruit-flavored	1 cup	227	10	2.6	42.3	193
Big Mac hamburger	1 burger	570	24.6	35	39.2	472

GAME MEAT

Sure this seems pretty exotic and expensive, but, hey, if dining is entertainment, what could be more amusing and healthy than game meat? Harvey Hilderbran, executive director of the Exotic Wildlife Association, says sales of all game meat is on the rise. In 1983, $53,000 worth of venison was sold in Texas. By 1994, that amount rose to over $2.3 million. Mr. Hilderbran believes that there's probably more demand than there is supply.

While domesticated animals such as farmed deer are taken to a conventional slaughterhouse where they are killed and processed as are cattle, sheep, and goats, ranched deer can only be harvested by taking a mobile slaughter facility and meat inspector to the field, where the animals are killed by shooting them with a high-powered rifle under the supervision of the meat inspector. The carcass is then processed inside the mobile facility to avoid any contamination of the meat. Mike Hughes, owner of Broken Arrow Ranch in Ingram, Texas, believes that the way he harvests animals is more humane than the way traditional meat is killed. "We shoot them once in the head and the animals do not suffer. They don't experience stress and it improves the quality of the meat."

Game meat has special benefits including:

- Lowering cholesterol: One study, conducted at the Lipid Research Clinic at George Washington University in Washington, D.C., found that when buffalo meat was substituted four times a week for lean beef, total cholesterol and LDL were reduced significantly, even after the participants had started with stable blood cholesterol levels. Additionally, Martin Marchello, Ph.D., professor of animal and range sciences at North Dakota State University, says there's never been a report of an allergic reaction to game meat.

- Low in fat: Game animals don't stay fast and agile by marbling their muscle in a feedlot. Game meat is generally an extremely lean meat, both low in fat and calories, because the animals are exceptionally fit. Wild game meat averages one-seventh the fat of domestic meat. If you compare South Texas antelope to regular ground beef you'll find that antelope has only 2 percent fat while beef has 26.55 percent. Even the extra-lean variety of beef has 17.06 percent fat. Dr. Marchello says, "Game meats are much leaner than are domestic meats. Today, our lifestyle is sedentary compared to years and years ago when we engaged in heavy physical activity. We no longer need the total calories that domesticated animals offer us. A real benefit is that when we consume game meats we're consuming natural products out in nature that are free of antibiotics, hormones, and most likely pesticides."

If you still think low-fat meat is an oxymoron, look at the table below. South Texas antelope has less fat than soybeans, low-fat milk, even some grains! Game is the kind of tough food that keeps your teeth sharp and strong. Remember that hunter-gatherers lived, and lived well, off wild game millennia before there were cereals, breads, pastas, or bagels.

- Higher-quality fats: Stearic acid is viewed as a healthy fatty acid, where palmitic is downright dangerous. The University of Alabama has found that all domestic farm animals such as poultry, pork, lamb, and beef have 1 part stearic acid to 4 parts palmitic acid — both saturated fats. Bison has only 1 part stearic acid to 1 part palmitic acid. Do the math and you'll see that with one-seventh less fat, that works out to 28 times less palmitic acid.

- Flavor: Robert Waggoner, executive chef at the Wild Boar Restaurant in Nashville, Tennessee, says he loves cooking wild game because of its incredible flavor and texture. He says, "It has a gamey flavor, kind of an earthy, aged flavor. Unlike domesticated meat, it doesn't have that simple taste that you know means its diet has been fixed." Game meat from free-ranging animals produces a more complex flavor than domesticated animals because of the variety of their diet.

Comparison of Game versus Supermarket Meats

Protein	Calories (per 6 oz. serving)	Percent Fat
SUPERMARKET MEATS		
Beef, ground	531	26.55
Beef, ground, lean	453	20.67
Beef, ground, extra-lean	401	17.06
Lamb	447	14.29
Turkey	371	11.23
Chicken	200	3.23
LOW-FAT GAME MEATS		
Sika venison	273	3.91
Blackbuck antelope	216	2.72
Axis venison	233	2.55
Nilgai antelope	210	2.21
South Texas antelope	189	2

OTHER GAME MEATS   Native Game, a distributor of wild meats located in Golden Valley, Minnesota, distributes buffalo, venison, antelope, caribou, wild boar, bear, rattlesnake, rabbit, wild game birds such as quail, pheasant, squab, and wild turkey . . . just to name a few. Penny Davis of Native Game says that the main appeal is the health benefits. She says, "My husband is a chef and I've tried all of the game meats. It's the only thing I eat now. Before I got into this business I ate chicken and beef, but once you get into game you don't go back. There's so little fat in game meat. I can't stand looking at beef now. The allure of beef in regards to the taste and smell of it is really the fat!"

Buffalo: Huts Hamburgers, in Austin, Texas, offers buffalo burgers. Although they're $1.75 more than a regular hamburger, Laurie Womble, Huts' manager, says people are willing to pay the difference because they like the meat so much. She says, "It's a much leaner, drier meat. We find that people are much more health conscious and really think it's a great choice." Ms. Womble estimates that 10 to 15 percent of sales are buffalo. I tried a buffalo diet in Cuser, South Dakota, last summer. Buffalo burgers taste terrific but aren't oozing with fat. A buffalo burger eaten at noon will be killing your appetite for half a day or longer.

WHERE TO BUY GAME MEATS   There are dozens of distributors or ranchers from whom to buy. Here is a short list of suppliers:
- Native Game, in Golden Valley, MN: 800-952-6321
- D'Artagnan in Jersey City, NJ: 800-DARTAGNAN
- Broken Arrow Ranch, in Ingram, TX: 800-962-4263
- Game Sales, Inc., in Loveland, CO: 800-729-2090
- Polarica, in San Francisco and New York 800-GAMEUSA
- Colorado Mountain Game, in Denver, CO: 800-738-2750
- Wild Game, Inc., in Huron, Chicago, IL: 312-278-1661

COOKING GAME MEAT: SAFETY   Any lean red meat requires special attention when cooking to avoid drying out the meat and toughening it. Tender cuts of venison and antelope should be cooked as little as possible to retain the highest level of moisture. Quick sautéing, grilling, or roasting is best for tender cuts such as loin, tenderloin, and leg muscles. Some people will overcook because of concerns about unknown bacteria, but venison and antelope are among the purest meats you can prepare, offering little risk of danger from undercooking. Overcooking also dries out the meat and will make the texture more like that of liver. Braising is the best method for the other cuts of meat such as shoulder, ribs, and shanks. Safety: The FDA doesn't inspect raw meat; only the USDA does that. But game meat is not listed in either the Federal Meat Act or the Federal Poultry Act. Therefore, the USDA does not inspect game meat. Any game meat should be certified as inspected by either state or federal meat inspection authorities.

SOFT PROTEINS
These are proteins that are physically softened by processing or by the addition or presence of fats or carbohydrates.

NUTS
OK, you've got me on this one. Nuts are hard to bite into and chew on. So if I were fair, they would be hard foods. Right? Wrong. Most nuts are so high in fats that any official judge of hard foods would have to rule against them. However, in a truly all-hard-food, caveman diet, a few nuts are admissible as an added taste treat since they do crunch like hard foods on the back molars.

CANNED BEANS
Boiled to a pulp and then packed with bacon and pork in a heavy fat and sugar sauce, these beans uphold the image of a true trash food.

POWDERS
Protein powders reduce the hardest proteins to pumice. Removed is any necessity of tearing, grinding, chewing, or digesting these powders. While these are a wonderful way of getting extra protein into sick patients and body builders, they present a clear danger. When

combined with carbohydrates like glucose and malto dextrins, it becomes an engineered food that produces the highest insulin response possible. Yet, combined with a much more limited amount of carbohydrate, the protein can quickly pile tyrosine into the brain, making you alert and producing glucagon to lower your insulin level.

RED MEATS

Fatty red meat has been widely credited as a chief culprit in modern man's three leading causes of death: heart disease, stroke, and cancer. These meats are first softened by the marbling process where the animals stock up on mega-grain feeds in a stockyard, where they get little exercise. If you enjoy lots of red meat and are inactive, remember that you're becoming as well marbled as the beef you eat. Beef is further softened by grinding it into hamburger meat, cutting down on the work required by your teeth and digestive system. This is the same principle we looked at with carbohydrates: Make the food particles smaller in size and make them softer to speed their digestion.

SOFT DAIRY

Butter, whole milk, and fatty cheeses cost a frightening price in added calories and fat. But the stealth category here is the frozen yogurt or milkshake. Low-fat yogurts are often sugar-softened foods with nearly 30 grams of added sugars. That softening adds a tremendous number of calories, a desire to overeat, and terrific potentiators for fattening you.

CALORIE COST OF PROTEINS: THE SAFETY ISSUE

The doom-and-gloom crowd claims that too much protein causes kidney failure and washes calcium out of bone to cause osteoporosis. They have solid backing in the scientific community. Dr. Walter Willett of Harvard's School of Public Health believes there are legitimate concerns about calcium loss on a high-protein diet. Walter speculates that animal proteins are a much more likely villain than plant proteins. However, the kidney-failure issue is circumstantial. Patients who already have kidney damage will deteriorate faster on a high-protein diet than a low-protein one. Populations that eat higher amounts of protein have a higher rate of kidney failure than those that eat low amounts. One very likely reason that too much protein may lead to kidney failure is that high-fat, high-salt animal proteins may lead to hypertension and diabetes, two key precursors for kidney disease. That makes it difficult to tease out the root cause. Is it the protein itself, or is it the high amount of animal fat and salt that can come with it? Medical anthropologists point to late Paleolithic man, who ate 33 percent of his calories as protein but still enjoyed robust health until being run down by a wild animal. But these anthropologists are quite certain that Paleolithic man didn't develop diabetes or hypertension. On that basis they believe that the combination of vegetable and extremely lean animal proteins is unlikely to be dangerous if you stay within the limits recommended above. So how much is too much? The real safety issue has been obscured by both the more-protein crowd and the old school nutritionists. "High" protein is described as a 30 percent protein diet; "normal" protein is a 12 percent protein diet. But this misrepresents the issue. If you successfully use the satiating effects of protein to eat fewer calories, you could end up eating fewer grams of protein than you do now, but have a higher percent of protein in your diet. Let's look at the math. If you eat a 30 percent fat diet and your calories total out at 5,000, you will be eating 375 grams of protein. That is clearly off the top end of anyone's safety charts. But 30 percent of 1,500 calories, or 113 grams, is a safe and effective amount for an active 200-pound man. So rather than picking the percent protein you plan to eat, use protein before a meal as a satiator, but keep the total number of grams within the safe limits outlined in Step Two (on page 102).

If you want to eat less protein and still get all its benefits, stick to proteins with a very high biological value (BV). BV is calculated by the efficiency with which muscles can take up and use protein to become larger. According to Frank Katch, Ph.D., the biologic value of food refers to the completeness with which it supplies essential amino acids. High-quality protein foods are of animal origin, whereas vegetables are incomplete in terms of one or more essential amino acids and thus have a low BV. However, all of the essential amino acids can be obtained by consuming a variety of plant foods — grains, fruits, and vegetables. The key for high BV is not to pig out on fatty animal meats but to combine grains and legumes!! Dr. Peter Lemon of Kent State University says, "The BV is based on the amount of a nutrient that is actually absorbed from the human intestine. So if you have a high BV protein that means that it has been measured in humans and a higher percentage of the nutrients are actually retained by the human as opposed to excreted. So, it's really a direct measure of the value."

Penn State's Dr. Bill Evans says, "Let's assume you're consuming a low biological value protein; only 80 percent of it is retained (to make new muscle). If you consume a high biological value protein you can assume that 95 percent of it will be retained. You get more bang for your buck by eating high biological protein. The issue is not whether the protein is vegetable or meat protein but whether it is high or low. For example, soy protein is a very high BV whereas some other vegetable protein is much lower. But the same rule applies." By eating high-quality protein, you can eat 16 percent less protein than the low-quality variety and still get the same nutrient value.

Hard Fibers

Fibers have the most powerful positive effects on hunger control known. The higher your fiber and the lower your glucose load, the better control you have over your insulin and your weight. The lower your fiber and higher your glucose load, the higher your insulin and the more difficult your weight will be to control.

Conventional Wisdom
Refined foods.

LEAN
High-fiber foods.

ROAD MAP
This chapter pulls together all you've heard about fiber so far in this book. There are extensive lists of those foods highest in fiber.

BACKGROUND
Doctors Denis Burkitt and Hugh Trowell first developed the dietary fiber hypothesis, theorizing that a diet rich in foods that contain fiber is protective against obesity. They believed that a high-fiber diet derived from whole grain cereal, legumes, fruits, and vegetables could lead to the remission of many diseases through fiber's effect on blood glucose control, cholesterol, blood pressure, and body fat. In 1945, Dr. Alex Walker noticed that black South Africans from rural homelands had a lower incidence of certain gastrointestinal and metabolic disorders than did urban black and Caucasian people. He thought this was due to the differences in the consumption of dietary fiber.

Dr. Trowell linked the bulky stools of Africans to high-fiber intake and the low prevalence of Western diseases.

Those theories moved into the laboratory in 1961 when researchers reported on the beneficial metabolic effects of the individual components of fiber: pectin and guar. Dr. Ancel Keys demonstrated that pectin intake decreased serum cholesterol; Dr. David Jenkins later reported that guar and pectin decreased the rise in blood glucose following a meal; and Dr. James Anderson reported that high-fiber diets lowered insulin and medication requirements for people with all forms of diabetes and helped them lose weight.

FOODS TO CHOOSE FOR WEIGHT CONTROL AND HUNGER-CUTTING FOODS

HIGH-SOLUBLE-FIBER FOODS

The best single marker of a hard food is the amount of soluble fiber, the hardest of hard-core fibers. Studies by James W. Anderson, M.D., professor of medicine and clinical nutrition at the University of Kentucky College of Medicine and chief of the endocrinology metabolic section at the Veterans Affairs Medical Center in Lexington, Kentucky, show that soluble fiber slows gastric emptying and decreases mixing of foods and digestive enzymes in the small intestine. Hard fibers are the most potent single component of foods when it comes to killing hunger, lowering insulin, and decreasing risk of heart disease. These are the direct effects of soluble fiber:

- provides less energy-dense food
- increases satiety
- decreases glucose and insulin after a meal
- increases muscle sensitivity to insulin so less insulin is necessary
- slows the rate of fat absorption
- increases bile excretion, which dumps fats from the body
- decreases the manufacture of new fats in the liver

Pretty potent stuff, but make no mistake about it, foods containing hard fibers are far and few between. You will hear many people complain that they don't get the full effects of fiber, but if you examine the foods they eat, you will find few soluble fibers in them. To qualify as a hard-fiber food, it must be high in soluble fiber and low in its glucose load. The following table lists those foods with the highest amount of soluble fiber. The table is constructed to show you how many grams of soluble fiber are in roughly 400 calories of food. The foods which lead the list pack the most fiber per calorie to give you the biggest bang for the buck. If you are on a very-limited-calorie diet, say 1,000–1,500 calories, pick most of your carbohydrate calories from these high-fiber foods. (Oatmeal is listed as uncooked because the degree of cooking has a highly variable result on the final fiber amount.)

When you shop for these foods, be certain that they don't contain more than 5 grams of sugar per serving and that they don't contain saturated or hydrogenated fats, all of which cancel the weight-loss and health properties of fiber. From a purely practical standpoint, you'll find beans and high-fiber breakfast cereals to be the most reasonable way to eat large quantities of soluble fiber. Otherwise you're faced with eating huge amounts of vegetables or grains. For instance, you would need 1,600 calories of brussels sprouts, well beyond hard core, to get 10 grams of soluble fiber. That's not to discount vegetables, which should be eaten for their bulk, mineral, vitamin, antioxidant, and phytochemical values. Contrast that to Heartwise cereal with over 10 grams in a bowl . . . pretty amazing stuff.

As long as white flours, hydrogenated oils, and added sugars are absent, cereals are the second most efficient source of fiber. But be warned that many cereals are still heavily processed foods and contain high glucose loads. Note too that strikingly few grains make the grade. My favorite of those that do is really good pumpernickel bread such as Mestemacher's.

Beware that good hard soluble-fiber foods can be wrecked by overcooking. I like to slightly undercook grains, beans, and veggies. Here's an example: Whole wheat uncooked macaroni has 2.1 grams of soluble fiber, but after cooking it limps in with only 0.6 grams. Be sure to read the label as well. Fiber One, as an example, has an astounding 13 grams of fiber in a single serving, but that is not all naturally occurring fiber — some is from guar, which is an added fiber. Fiber researchers at Harvard feel strongly that the fiber should come from real foods because those foods have antioxidant minerals, vita-

High-Soluble-Fiber Foods

Food (400-calorie serving)	Soluble Fiber (grams)
CEREAL	
Oat Bran Crunch	9.3
oat bran and oat germ	7.6
Oat bran cereal, cold	5.2
All bran	5.1
Oat bran cereal, hot	4.8
Crispy oats	4.5
Fruit and Fitness	4.2
Cheerios	4.2
Common Sense	4.1
Oat flakes	3.6
Real oat bran cereal	3.5
Puffed wheat	3.4
All bran with extra fiber	3.2
Grapenuts	3
Fiber One	3
Quaker Oats squares	2.9
Oat bran flakes	2.7
Oat Bran O's	2.6
Nutri Grain	2.5
Wheaties	2.4
Raisin bran	2.4
Total whole wheat	2.2
Shredded wheat and bran	2.2
Wheat flakes	2
GRAINS	
Oat four	5.5
rye flour	3.9
Pearl uncooked barley	3.4
Wheat bran	3.4
Wheat germ	3.2
Whole wheat flour	1.8
BREADS	
Pumpernickel bread	3.9
Rye bread	3

High-Soluble-Fiber Foods

Food (400-calorie serving)	Soluble Fiber (grams)
FRUITS	
Dried apricots	4.4
Dried figs	4
Dried prunes	3.8
Dried peaches	3.8
VEGETABLES	
Okra pods, fresh, trimmed	2.9
Parsley, fresh	2.8
Brussels sprouts, fresh, cooked	2.5
Turnip, cooked	2.2
Cabbage, winter savoy, fresh	2
LEGUMES	
Kidney beans, dark red, dried, cooked	3.2
Cranberry beans, dried, cooked	3.1
Butter beans, dried, cooked	2.9
Black beans, cooked	2.8
Navy beans, dried, cooked	2.4
Pinto beans, dried, cooked	2.2
NUTS AND SEEDS	
Filberts (hazelnuts)	2.5
Sunflower seeds	2.1
BAKERY GOODS	
Oat bran animal cookies	2.5
Oat bran fancy fruit muffin	2.4
Oat bran fruit jumbo cookies	2.4
Oat bran fruit and nut cookies	2

This table is reprinted with permission from the HCF Nutrition Research Foundation, Inc.

mins, and other healthy components. Ten grams is about all most Americans' digestive systems can tolerate in the first week of eating a high soluble-fiber diet, without suffering excess gas or intestinal discomfort.

HIGH-INSOLUBLE-FIBER FOODS

While soluble fiber interacts with the digestive fluids and sops up water to fill you up, insoluble has a less powerful effect on weight control. Insoluble does control weight by providing a feeling of fullness and accelerating the passage of food into the colon, which decreases the time available to digest food. That leaves some food undigested, so you can enjoy eating it but not suffer the caloric consequences. Harvard's Dr. Eric Rimm confirms that insoluble fiber cuts hunger by improving satiety. If you choose to go the hard-core route and get your fiber through soluble-fiber foods, you needn't continue reading — you've got all the fiber you need. That's because for every gram of soluble fiber in a food, there are usually another 3 grams of insoluble fiber. If, however, you look at the high-soluble-fiber table above and say "No way," insoluble fibers are a great alternative; you'll just have to eat a great deal more of them. There's an added bonus. New evidence from the Harvard School of Public Health shows that insoluble fiber has an astounding effect on your risk of heart disease. For every extra gram you eat each day, your risk of heart disease decreases by 2 percent. Beware that many insoluble-fiber foods that lack soluble fiber, such as white flour bagels, English muffins, waffles, and pancakes, have a high glucose load. Remember to look at the FDA food label for total fiber over 5 grams per serving and sugars less than 5 grams, with no white flour, the "5-and-5 rule." The foods in the following table contain the highest amounts of insoluble fiber. The real surprises are fruits, vegetables, and beans. The veggies and fruits have very little insoluble fiber; their real strength weighs in with the heavier-duty soluble fibers. The same is true for over half the beans on the list. But for beans, the high amount of powerful soluble fibers far outweighs any deficit of insoluble fiber. The cutoff to qualify as a "high" insoluble-fiber food is 9 grams per 400 calories. That way, on

Insoluble Fiber per 400 Calories of Each Food

Food	Insoluble fiber (grams)
CEREALS	
All Bran with Extra Fiber	46.20
Fiber One	39.40
All Bran	25.70
40% Bran Flakes	13.80
Fruit and Fitness	11.10
Raisin Bran	11.10
Shredded Wheat	10.90
Heartwise	9.80
GRAINS	
Corn bran, uncooked	80.40
Wheat bran	37.60
Wheat germ	14.30
Popcorn, popped	10.80
Flour, whole wheat	9.10
Flour, rye	9.00
Barley, pearl, uncooked	8.40
Spaghetti, whole wheat, uncooked	7.80
Macaroni, whole wheat, uncooked	6.90
Cornmeal, blue	6.90
Oatmeal, uncooked	4.60
Flour, oat	4.00
BREADS AND CRACKERS	
Bread, mixed grain "lite"	12.70
Crackers, snack, whole wheat	9.10
Bread, cellulose	8.80
Melba toast, wheat	7.10
Bread, rye (German)	6.80
Bread, pumpernickel	4.50
Bread, rye	3.60
FRUITS	
Peaches, dried	4.20
Figs, dried	4.20
Apricots, dried	3.50
Prunes, dried	2.80
VEGETABLES	
Okra pods, fresh, trimmed	4.40
Turnip, cooked	3.90

Insoluble Fiber per 400 Calories of Each Food

Food	Insoluble fiber (grams)
Brussels sprouts, fresh	2.70
Parsley, fresh	2.60
Brussels sprouts, cooked	2.40
Parsnip, cooked	1.90
Cabbage, winter savoy, fresh	1.80
Celeriac, fresh	1.60
LEGUMES	
White beans, Great Northern, dried, uncooked	13.30
Pinto beans, dried, uncooked	11.90
Kidney beans, dark red, dried, uncooked	11.30
Butter beans, dried, uncooked	10.60
Soybeans, dried, uncooked	10.50
Lentils, dried, uncooked	10.30
Chickpeas, dried, uncooked	8.50
Mung beans, dried, uncooked	8.20
Split beans, dried, uncooked	5.10
Pinto beans, dried, cooked	4.70
Navy beans, dried, cooked	4.70
Kidney beans, dark red, dried, cooked	4.60
Butter beans, dried, cooked	4.40
Black beans, cooked	4.30
Cranberry beans, dried, cooked	3.00
Pork and beans with sauce, cooked	2.20
NUTS AND SEEDS	
Coconut, dried	14.90
Almonds	7.70
Coconut, fresh	7.70
Sesame seeds	7.20
Filberts (hazelnuts)	5.20
Peanuts, fresh	5.10
Peanuts, roasted	5.10
Sunflower seeds	4.00

Insoluble Fiber per 400 Calories of Each Food	
Food	Insoluble fiber (grams)
HEALTH FOOD	
Oat Bran Graham Cookies	5.60
Oat Bran Fruit Jumbo Cookies	5.20
Oat Bran Animal Cookies	5.00
Oat Bran Fruit and Nut Cookies	4.00
Oat Bran Fancy Fruit Muffin	3.60

Insoluble Fiber per 400 Calories of Each Food	
Food	Insoluble fiber (grams)
Oat Bran Jumbo Fruit Bar	3.10
Oat bran raisin muffin	2.60

Table adapted with permission from HCF Nutrition Research Foundation, Inc.

a 2,000-calorie-a-day diet, you'd get just 35 grams of fiber if all your carbohydrates contained the minimum 9 grams of fiber per 400 calories. The table shows the amount of insoluble fiber found in 400 calories of food ranked from highest to lowest for cereals, grains, breads, fruits, vegetables, legumes, nuts and seeds. Foods in italics are not high in insoluble fiber but are listed for demonstration purposes.

HOW TO USE FIBER

- Before meals: Fiber acts as a super appetite killer that quiets hunger to allow you to choose a far leaner meal.
- As a snack: Holds over through the next meal so you make great choices.
- As a meal: The best way to decrease your glucose load and extra fat.

Hard Beans

Beans have gotten a bad rap from the time we were kids spouting the ditty "Beans, beans, . . . the more you eat the more you toot." What you may not recall from grade school is that the verse continues: "the more you toot the better you feel, so eat your beans at every meal." If you did eat beans at every meal you would feel awesome. Beans deliver an astonishing array of tastes, textures, health benefits, and positive alterations in mood chemistry. The mistake we made as kids was assuming that those brown beans canned in lard that made us toot had the same nutritional value as well-prepared, carefully selected super beans.

Conventional Wisdom
Beans make you toot.

LEAN
God has already given us designer foods. They're called beans.

Beans are a footnote in most American diets. They're discounted as a major source of protein and viewed simply as another unpalatable vegetable. Yet beans have tremendous virtues as a dieter's delight, killing your hunger for hours while lowering your blood sugar, insulin, and cholesterol levels. Why haven't you heard more about beans? Beans are a very cheap commodity for which there hasn't been much impetus to market or conduct research. Belinda Smith, M.S., R.D., L.D., a University of Kentucky research associate, says beans are pennies per pound. "They're a great, cheap source of protein. They add texture and heartiness to meatless meals when you combine them with a grain," she says. I consider beans the missing food group. Most of us think of beans as overcooked slop. Properly cooked beans taste great.

ROAD MAP

This chapter has great lists for the best beans, including those with the most soluble fiber, the lowest glycemic index, the most tyrosine and nutrients. It also gives you all the steps you need to deal with gas. You'll notice that not every bean is in every table in this chapter, since research comes from different institutions that made different choices of beans to study, so make your selection based on the effect you are looking for. First choose high-soluble-fiber beans to kill your hunger and low-GI beans to cut your insulin level. Then look for high-tyrosine beans to energize yourself and high-nutrient beans to balance your diet. The end of the chapter discusses super beans that have the most powerful and greatest array of health benefits of any foods known.

BENEFITS

HUNGER-CUTTING PROTEIN Most experts believe that plant proteins in beans are safe at the higher protein consumptions necessary to cut hunger. Here's why. A bean diet counters the two highest risks of a high-protein diet: the diabetes and hypertension that can lead to kidney failure. The calcium washed out by high-protein diets is replaced by the calcium in beans. Soybeans, as you'll read, actually prevent osteoporosis. If you're really going to bulk up on protein, beans are the way to do it safely.

INCREASED SATIETY Fiber foods require a great deal of chewing and take a lot of time to eat. Beans are a bulky food which fills you up on a very limited number of calories. Once you drink several glasses of water, the soluble fiber fills you up.

CUT BLOOD FAT Studies have shown that as little as one half to one cup of beans per day can significantly reduce blood cholesterol and control blood sugar in patients with diabetes. University of Kentucky's Dr. James W. Anderson's long-term studies indicate that the daily intake of 50 grams of beans can substantially reduce serum cholesterol levels and actually increase serum HDL-cholesterol levels.

CUT BLOOD SUGAR   Belinda Smith, M.S., R.D., L.D., puts it all together nicely when she says, "The soluble fiber in beans, which gels in the intestine, is great for a slow rise in blood sugar. It slows the process of glucose going into the cell. It lowers the rise in glucose. Once you lower the amount of blood sugar in the blood, you need less insulin to control the blood sugar."

BEANS FOR WEIGHT CONTROL
HUNGER-CUTTING BEANS
Beans are the richest single source of soluble fiber, the ultimate weight-loss fiber, with pinto beans topping the list. Here's how beans are ranked for soluble-fiber content. Look carefully at the table and you'll see that uncooked pinto beans have 7.5 grams of soluble fiber where cooked pinto beans only have 2.2 grams. That shows the enormous softening power of boiling beans for long periods.

BEANS THAT LOWER BLOOD SUGAR   Beans are the richest available source of the slow-release factors to lower insulin, blood sugar, and cholesterol levels. Beans have the lowest glycemic index of any group

Soluble Fiber in Beans

Beans	Soluble Fiber (per 100 grams)
Pinto beans, dried, uncooked	7.5
Kidney beans, dark red, dried, uncooked	6.9
Soybeans, dried, uncooked	6.8
Butter beans, dried, uncooked	6.3
White beans, Great Northern, dried, uncooked	4.4
Chickpeas, dried, uncooked	3.3
Kidney beans, dark red, dried, cooked	3.2
Cranberry beans, dried, cooked	3.1
Butter beans, dried, cooked	2.9
Black beans, cooked	2.8
Mung beans, dried, uncooked	2.8
Navy beans, dried, cooked	2.4
Pinto beans, dried, cooked	2.2
Split beans, dried, uncooked	2.2
Pork and beans with sauce, canned	2
Lentils, dried, uncooked	1.2

Table adapted with permission from HCF Nutrition Research Foundation, Inc.

of foods, which best reflects their slow-release nature. Here's a ranking of glycemic index values for a variety of beans. Soybeans top the list at 15. Beans with a GI in the 20s are still terrific. Over 40, however, gives them nearly triple the glucose-raising action of soybeans.

BEANS THAT ENERGIZE   Beans contain high levels of the amino acid tyrosine, sufficient to increase the blood levels of tyrosine, which is required for dopamine synthesis in the brain. A rise in brain dopamine leads to increased vigor and energy and increases your concentration while simultaneously cutting stress.

To get a sense of just how good a source beans are, look at the second table on page 128, where soybeans outdistance beef, chicken, or fish by nearly five to one.

MOST NUTRITIOUS BEANS
Only a few vegetables rank higher for nutrients than beans — and beans outrank even the best grains by four to one. If you're not keen on a plateful of veggies, beans are a great way to pick up the slack.

Glycemic Index for Beans

Beans	Glycemic Index
Soybeans, boiled	15
South African brown beans	24
Mesquite flour	25
Red beans	26
Kidney beans	27
Lentils	29
Yellow teparies broth	29
Green beans	30
Mexican black beans	30
Tepary beans	30
Butter beans	31
White teparies broth	31
Lima beans, baby, frozen	32
Split peas, yellow, boiled	32
Black-eyed peas	33
Chickpeas	33

Glycemic Index for Beans

Beans	Glycemic Index
Garbanzo/chickpeas	36
Lima beans, broth	36
Haricot (navy) beans	38
Mexican brown beans	38
Pinto beans	39
Black-eyed beans	42
Pinto beans, canned	45
Romano beans	46
Peas	47
Baked beans	48
Green beans, canned	52
Broad beans	79

Table adapted with permission from the *American Journal of Clinical Nutrition* 62 (1995): 871–935.

Tyrosine Levels of Beans

Beans (1 cup cooked)	Tyrosine (grams)
Soybeans	2.50
Split peas	1.40
Mung beans	0.54
Butter beans	0.51
Adzuki	0.51
Lentils	0.48
Great Northern	0.47
Kidney beans, dark red	0.45
Navy beans	0.44
Black-eyed peas	0.43
Black beans	0.43
Pink beans	0.43
Pinto beans	0.39
Garbanzo beans (canned)	0.36
Lima beans	0.33

Information provided by Belinda Smith, M.S., R.D., L.D.

Beans deliver a powerhouse of minerals and vitamins as a nearly complete meal all on their own. The table opposite shows how they rank.

GAS

I look at beans, more than any other food in this book, as powerful medicines that solidly deliver all the important weight-control functions of foods. Rather than trying to figure out how to make bean dishes, just aim at eating ⅓ to 1 cup of beans three times a day. It's that simple. The limiting factors for beans are preparation time and passing gas. Passing gas may seem like a large price to pay, but it is due to the soluble fiber in beans, which is the single most powerful weight-control factor that occurs in foods.

Tyrosine Comparison Table

Protein	Tyrosine
Soybeans, 1 cup cooked	2.50 grams
Beef (2 oz.)	0.47 grams
Chicken (2 oz.)	0.59 grams
Fish (2 oz.)	0.49 grams
Egg (1)	0.25 grams

CSPI Food Value of Beans

Beans (1 cup cooked)	SCORE
Soybeans	300
Pinto beans	287
Chickpeas (garbanzos, ceci)	286
Lentils	285
Cranberry beans	278
Black-eyed peas (cowpeas)	273
Pink beans	269
Navy beans	266
Black beans (turtle beans)	265
Small white beans	263
White beans	253
Lima beans, baby	252
Kidney beans, all types	243
Adzuki beans	238
Great Northern beans	228
Mung beans	226
Lima beans, large	224
Broad beans (fava beans)	197

CSPI Food Value of Beans

Beans (1 cup cooked)	SCORE
Peas, split (green)	192
Tofu, raw, firm (4 oz.)	178
Tofu, raw, regular	109

Center for Science in the Public Interest came up with a score for each bean by adding its percent of the U.S. Recommended Daily Allowance (USRDA) for seven nutrients (folic acid, magnesium, iron, copper, zinc, protein, and vitamin B) plus fiber and potassium. There are no USRDA's for fiber or potassium so they used the Daily Value of 25 grams for fiber and their own RDA of 3,500 milligrams for potassium. Copyright 1993, CSPI. Reprinted and adapted from *Nutrition Action Healthletter* (1875 Connecticut Ave. N.W., Suite 300, Washington, D.C. 20009-5728; $24.00 for 10 issues).

The Roman emperor Claudius declared, "All citizens shall be allowed to pass gas whenever necessary." According to a new survey, Americans are less embarrassed about passing gas than they used to be. The survey, conducted by Block Drug Company, Inc., found that while 75 percent of respondents admit they pass gas at least once a week and almost one-third pass gas daily, 44 percent of all respondents say they are not embarrassed. However, the very prospect of farting so overwhelms some of those who would be the thinnest that millions avoid beans to avoid embarrassment. Don't! You'll find that your body does adjust very nicely to beans and the gas problem disappears. Hard-core vegetarians, like the employees of the Pritikin Longevity Center in Santa Monica, California, claim to be completely gas-free bean eaters. But that transition period is one most Americans don't have the patience to tough out. The reason so few people make the transition to daily bean consumption is that there is explosive and noisy warfare in the gut between the good new bacteria that beans introduce and the bad old bacteria that don't want to depart. Flatulence is caused by a buildup of gas in the large intestine.

The gas is formed as a result of the action of bacteria on carbohydrates and amino acids in digested foods. Air swallowing and foods are the primary culprits. Eating quickly is the surest way to create gas. Technically speaking, a small amount of the carbohydrate in beans is from certain sugars that cause most of the intestinal problems. Our stomachs do not contain the enzymes required to digest these sugars. They therefore arrive undigested in the large intestine. Bacteria that live in the large intestine readily feed off of and ferment the sugars, producing carbon dioxide, hydrogen, and a few other gases that all add up to flatulence. The sugars responsible for gas production, called fructo-oligo saccharides in soybeans, are associated with great health benefits. These sugars are nondigestible, leaving only bacteria to feed on them and, in turn, produce gas. Doctors once thought they were useless, but now know that these good bacteria act as scavengers. They clean up the intestine and suppress the bad bacteria, called clostridia. Once the war is won, your gut should settle down. Part of the gas from beans is caused by increasing the fiber content of your diet. If you gradually do so, your body will adapt to the change and your discomfort will diminish.

HOW TO AVOID GAS

- Don't gulp food or beverages.
- Avoid eating hard candies, smoking, and drinking carbonated drinks if you have a gas problem. They all increase air swallowing, which increases intestinal gas.
- Choose "gas light" beans such as pintos, lentils, and garbanzos over white beans.
- Start slowly. If you were put on an antidepressant, you would be given ever larger doses over a two-week period. The same is true with beans: You need to start slowly — one-quarter cup a day in week one, then a half a cup, working your way up to as much as two cups a day over the course of six weeks. If you have a high risk of diabetes or are trying to prevent diabetes, work your way up to three cups a day.
- Use fresh beans.

- Soak beans thoroughly; soak overnight and pour off water. Chris Kilham, author of *The Bread & Circus Whole Food Bible,* recommends the following method to reduce the gas-producing effects of beans: Soak the beans, pouring off the soaking water, and cooking the beans in fresh water. My most knowledgeable food friend, Lindsay Herkness, changes the water ten times during the soaking phase to eliminate gas.
- Eat small, frequent meals.
- Boil for ten minutes and pour off foam before cooking.
- Chew thoroughly.

BEAN RELIEF PRODUCTS

Beano (Akpharma, Inc.)

Beano improves the digestibility of gassy food like beans, broccoli, cabbage, and peas. Beano tablets or drops contain a natural food enzyme, alphagalactosidase, which breaks down the complex sugars found in gassy foods into simple sugars our body can digest, making them less likely to cause bloating and flatulence. The company claims to receive over four thousand calls per week on their hotline, 800-257-8650. Beano is offered at Dr. Dean Ornish's programs in addition to other wellness retreats, health food stores, supermarkets, and pharmacies throughout the country.

Phazyme Gas Relief (Block Drug Company, Inc.)

This product is an antiflatulent medication containing simethicone, an agent proven to relieve gas. Phazyme works by altering the activity of small gas bubbles in the large intestine. In addition, simethicone relieves gas by dispersing and preventing further formation of gas pockets in the intestine.

HOW TO USE BEANS

BEFORE A MEAL

High-soluble-fiber beans taken before a meal are a great filler. After you've eaten them, take several glasses of water; that will expand the beans to fill your stomach. This technique also gets more tyrosine to your brain to make more alerting neurotransmitters.

AS AN APPETIZER

A good black bean soup or bean salad serves as a great filler if you have to suffer through a restaurant meal.

AS A MAIN COURSE

Bean/grain combinations are the lifeblood of thousands of cultures around the world. Combined with the right whole grains, you have a complete meal, such as black beans and brown rice. The chapter "Beans and Grains" lists lots more.

AS A SNACK MEAL

Soy nuts provide an almost complete meal. A soy snack will fill you up and give you the alerting hit of a good protein.

SUPER BEANS

THE SOYBEAN

I always knew soy was good for you but I never knew just how good until I finished researching this book. Imagine a food that energizes you while it cuts stress, lowers the risk of many diseases, and helps control your weight. Wow! Here are the reasons soy has become the world's premier superfood.

Breast and Prostate Cancer Prevention

Dr. Ken Setchell of the Cincinnati Children's Hospital Medical Center has shown that women eating a soy diet for one month change their menstrual cycles to match those of Asian women, who have lower rates of breast cancer. As an antitumor agent against breast cancer, soy protein or soy isoflavones — the active ingredient in soybeans — inhibit the development of breast (and prostate) cancer. Isoflavones are thought to inhibit a number of adverse reactions and act as antioxidants. Dr. Setchell says soy has virtually the same potent antiestrogen effects as seen with the anticancer drug tamoxifen. Genistein, a major soy isoflavone, also inhibits growth of a number of cancer cells in laboratory tests and inhibits new blood vessel growth that is essential for tumor cell growth. UCLA is running a large prostate cancer prevention program using soy protein. One well-known participant is Mike Milken. The NCI is also funding trials to prevent the recurrence of breast cancer.

Cholesterol Lowering

The *New York Times* called soybeans "among the most potent cholesterol-lowering dietary factors yet discovered." Of his classic *New England Journal of Medicine* review of soy research, University of Kentucky's Dr. James Anderson says, "Our study indicated that consuming 17 to 25 grams of soy protein per day could have meaningful effects on serum cholesterol levels. Soy protein intake was associated with a 9.3 percent reduction in serum cholesterol, a 12.9 percent reduction in serum LDL-cholesterol and a 10.5 percent reduction in serum triglycerides. HDL-cholesterol (the good kind) levels increased by 2.4 percent."

Great Source of Fiber

Soy fiber has double the dietary fiber of whole wheat.

Great Source of Protein

Soy is 38 percent protein, double the content of many meats. The protein in soy supplies all essential amino acid needs for human health. On one scale of protein values, it outranks every other edible source of protein.

Great Source of Essential Fatty Acids

Soybeans contain the essential fatty acid, linoleic acid, from which the body makes its own heart protective Omega 3 fatty acids. Experts like Dr. Anderson say soy has antioxidant properties that protect LDL from the oxidation that causes blockages in the coronary arteries. He also says that both men and women can benefit from as little as 25 grams of soy protein each day, which could reduce serum cholesterol levels by about 7 to 10 percent and lower the risk for heart disease by 15 to 25 percent.

Osteoporosis Prevention

Soy isoflavones act much like the antiestrogen tamoxifen, which reduces the risk for osteoporosis. Epidemiologic studies show that vegetarian women who have higher intakes of soy protein have lower
rates of osteoporosis. Since substantial weight loss from dieting in
women can lead to osteoporosis, soy is an important dieter's food.

Endurance

Soy is a rich source of choline, which MIT's Richard Wurtman has
intensively investigated. Choline is the precursor for the neurotransmitter acetylcholine. About ten years ago his group from MIT collected blood samples of runners before and after the Boston
Marathon. They discovered that choline levels had dropped about 40
percent over the course of the twenty-six miles. Swimmers who took
choline supplements were able to swim longer without muscle fatigue. So soy can help give you the endurance to sweat off those extra pounds.

Low Glycemic Index

Soybeans set the record for slow-burning foods. They have the lowest recorded glycemic index value of any foods tested by Native
Seeds. Their GI index is 15. That makes oatmeal, at 49, look like a
hot fudge sundae. Soybeans are so low that the occasional dietary in-
discretion is much more easily tolerated if you've eaten soy.

Soy-Containing Foods

Soy protein products are widely available today. Soy beverages, tofus,
textured soy protein, isolated soy protein, and soy flour can be used as
foods or put in main dishes and bakery products. Tofu is a wonderful
soy protein product. It was first used in China around 200 B.C. It is
made from soybeans, which are washed, soaked, drained, ground,
cooked in a soy slurry, and put through a soy milk extraction. A co-
agulant is added, the product is pressed, the tofu block is cut, and it is
packaged, sealed, pasteurized, packed in cases, and put in cold storage. There are several types of tofu. Firm, which is dense and solid,
works well in stir-fry dishes, soups, or on the grill. It is also the type

that is highest in protein, fat, and calcium than the other forms. Soft is good for recipes with blended tofu. Silken, which is a creamy, custardlike product, works well in blended and pureed dishes.

Soy Foods That Taste Great

The first and second generation of soy foods flopped because they just didn't taste good. Most Americans failed to adapt to the traditional soy foods: soy milk, tofu, tempeh, and miso. In fact, Johanna H. Dwyer, director of the Frances Stern Nutrition Center in Boston, found many women simply unwilling to eat large amounts of traditional soy foods even if they produced more favorable estrogen levels to prevent breast cancer. As a result, she couldn't recruit enough women to validate a four-year study she was undertaking. Third-generation soy products taste great and submerge the issue of poor aftertaste.

The new improved soyburger is my weekday lunch. I truly like these better than hamburgers going down and love them for their soothing aftereffects. These have a true burgerlike mouth feel and taste but without the heavy, pit-of-your-stomach aftereffect. It's a great quick-hit meal with lots of veggies and soy. The White House orders Boca Burgers, which have nearly zero fat. Boca Burgers, manufactured by the Boca Burger Co., in Fort Lauderdale, Florida, are tasty soyburgers that come in three different flavors. They can be found at supermarkets across the country.

Nuts: Soy is like the potato. Just as most of the potato's food value is in the skin, most of soy's mineral value is in the hull. Soy milk, which is usually de-hulled, then steamed and pressed, just doesn't have the same food value. The advantage of whole roasted soy nuts is that they retain the hull.

Soy shakes: The strong medical effects of soy include lowering cholesterol and reducing the chance of breast cancer. Soy protein powders are a superb source of super-high-quality protein. The soy shake is the easiest way to eat the huge amounts of soy necessary to protect you from prostate and breast cancer and to lower cholesterol. I add ice, some carbos, and water in a blender, then drink it like a milkshake. As a powder it's more quickly broken down and absorbed.

UCLA uses concentrated powders in its cancer-prevention trials. They know each subject is getting exactly enough. Soy protein powder is available as Vege Fuel from Twin Labs or directly from the manufacturer, Protein Technologies.

Engineered Foods: Look for soy-based muffins, breads, bakery items, shakes, soups, even pretzels that are engineered to taste great. Be sure to look at the label. Just because they have soy protein, doesn't mean they can't sneak in white flour or hydrogenated oils.

For more information on soy, you can contact the Soy Bean Council, a trade group, which has a consumer hotline for soy food information and recipes: 800-TALKSOY.

THE TEPARY BEAN   Traditionally, Native Americans were the top bean eaters. The Pima Indians were even nicknamed the "Bean People." In the summertime, Native Americans grew red beans, white and yellow tepary beans, black-eyed peas or cowpeas, and lima beans. In the winter they grew lentils, peas, and garbanzo beans or chickpeas. They got a major workout cultivating and collecting these foods. Desert Indians ate about 1½ cups of cultivated beans a day, in addition to wild beans like mesquite, which delivered huge quantities of slow-release factors. The tepary bean, however, is the most famous. Its name was derived from the Opata Indian word *tepar,* which means desert-adapted. Virtually no other cultivated beans can bear the intense 105-degree heat of the Sonoran Desert and still produce viable pollen and pods full of seeds. Their roots are known to reach twice as far down as those of common beans in the same amount of time, allowing them to tap deep reservoirs of soil moisture when upper layers have already dried. Whereas common beans continue to produce more seed with more water given to them, tepary seed yields peak out with a modest amount of soil moisture and decrease with overirrigation. They need a certain degree of stress to trigger all-out seed production or else they will simply continue to put on more foliage. Tepary beans are high in soluble fiber. They have high amounts of insulin-reducing pectin and are small in size, which limits their ability to release gas. They are available from Native Seeds/SEARCH at 602-327-9123.

THE MUNG BEAN   Mung beans rival soybeans for their health bene-fits, which from the isoflavones and phytoestrogens, prevent disease and create beneficial bacteria in the GI tract.

Since beans require complementary grains to become complete proteins, the following chapter is devoted to the hard grains that are great choices to round out your meal.

Hard Grains

You're best thinking of grains as pure glucose. That may seem unfair, given the tremendously healthful grains available, but recall the disastrous effect the agricultural revolution had on human health. Look around you at the catastrophic effect of the low-fat, high-carbo diet on waistlines around the world. Easily accessible grains introduced the possibility of huge glucose loads . . . loads high enough for the body to start manufacturing its own saturated fats . . . even on the lowest of low-fat diets. Grains are foods that require strong governors be placed on them. They must be hard foods, high in fiber, and have a low glucose load.

Conventional Wisdom
Grains are health foods.

LEAN
Soft grains are fat foods.

ROAD MAP
This chapter has lists for the best grains: hunger-cutting grains, grains that cut your blood sugar level, and the most nutritious grains. In planning your diet, first choose hunger grains, the grains that cut your blood sugar. Balance your diet out with high-nutrient grains. The end of the chapter discusses squishy grains, which will get you into trouble fast.

HUNGER-CUTTING GRAINS
HIGH-SOLUBLE FIBER

Grains are an overrated source of soluble fiber. Except for highly engineered breakfast cereals, you would be very hard pressed to eat large quantities of soluble fiber when eating grains. What you will discover in a trip through the bread, cereal, and cracker section of your local supermarket is an appalling lack of fiber. On most products you'll find labels that read from "less than 1" to "3 grams." That's the reason that so few grains are really good for you. Add high fiber to physical firmness and large size and you have a perfect grain. To preserve physical firmness, undercook your grains so they remain chewy. Here's a look at grains that have been rated highest for fiber. The list is divided into cereals, grains, breads, and crackers and ranked from highest amount of soluble fiber to lowest.

While you're reading through the following items, be sure to refer to the accompanying chart to see the actual recommended foods in each of the following categories.

Breakfast Cereals

Most of those boxes on your supermarket shelf are loaded with fast-burning carbos, with added sugar for taste. Follow the 5-and-5 rule: more than 5 grams of fiber, less than 5 grams of sugar per serving. Beware the hydrogenated fats. A better bet would be these super-high-fiber cereals.

Adding Sugar

If high-fiber, low-GI cereals seem like tasteless dreck or your hard-grained oatmeal tastes like slop and you would rather return to your Sugar Pops, listen to this: You can have the best of both worlds by adding whatever kind of sugar you like to your oatmeal. Dr. Bill Evans, of Penn State's Noll Physiologic Research Lab, tried it both ways: oats with sugar and without sugar. The surprising conclusion: The blood sugar levels go up about the same whether the oats have added sugar or not. Dr. Evans says, "If you have the sugar with oats or with something with a lot of soluble fiber, you won't have this huge

Soluble Fiber in Grains

Grain	Soluble Fiber (per 400 calories)
CEREALS	
Heartwise K.	10.5
Oat Bran Crunch	9.3
Oat bran and oat germ	7.6
Oat Bran, uncooked	7.2
Oat Bran, cereal, cold	5.2
All Bran	5.1
Oatmeal, uncooked	4.9
Oat Bran Hot Cereal, Apples & Cinnamon, uncooked	4.8
Crispy Oats	4.5
Cheerios	4.2
Fruit and Fitness	4.2
Common Sense K.	4.1
Oat Flakes	3.6
Real Oat Bran Cereal, Almond Crunch	3.5
Puffed Wheat	3.4
All Bran with Extra Fiber	3.2
Fiber One	3
Grapenuts	3
Oat Squares	2.9
Oat Bran Flakes	2.7
Oat Bran O's	2.6
Nutri Grain Wheat K.	2.5
Raisin Bran	2.4
Wheaties	2.4
Shredded Wheat & Bran	2.2
Total, Whole Wheat	2.2
Wheat Flakes	2

Soluble Fiber in Grains

Grain	Soluble Fiber (per 400 calories)
Shredded Wheat	1.6
40% Bran Flakes	1.5
GRAINS	
Flour, oat	5.5
Oatmeal, uncooked	4.9
Flour, rye	3.9
Barley, pearl, uncooked	3.4
Wheat bran	3.4
Wheat germ	3.2
Macaroni, whole wheat, uncooked	2.1
Flour, whole wheat	1.8
Spaghetti, whole wheat, uncooked	1.7
Corn bran, uncooked	1.1
Cornmeal, blue	0.9
Corn bran, uncooked	0.5
Popcorn, popped	0.5
BREADS AND CRACKERS	
Pumpernickel bread	3.9
Rye bread	3
Crackers, snack, whole wheat	1.8
Melba toast, wheat	1.8
Rye bread (German)	1.5
Cellulose bread	1.1
Mixed grain "lite" bread	0.9
Wheat lite bread	0.7
White lite bread	0.5

This table is reprinted with permission from the HCF Nutrition Research Foundation, Inc.

increase in blood sugar and therefore it's not going to hinder your performance. It's not going to be any worse than the same amount of carbohydrate without sugar; it's just going to taste better."

The cereals ranked highest in soluble fiber are those to which you can add sugar without fear. Whole grains, however, are the raw materials for a mountain of fiber. They'll live or die by how much sugar and fat manufacturers add to them.

LOW GLUCOSE LOAD

Few grains have ever been found that cut your blood sugar, which is why they contribute so heavily to glucose load. Below is the list of all grains considered to have a low or moderately low glucose load. Remember the scale goes from 0 to well over 100, so all of these are great foods. Tests have not been perfomed on all grains. For other safe bets, choose those grains highest in soluble fiber from the list on the opposite page.

HIGH IN NUTRIENTS

Whole grains are a reasonable source of minerals and vitamins but pale in comparison with vegetables, which can have 80 percent more of these essential nutrients. The table on the next page shows how the Washington, D.C.-based Center for Science in the Public Interest (CSPI) ranks grains for their fiber, mineral, and vitamin content. You'll notice that the highest score for a grain is 73, whereas the highest ranked vegetable is 461 and the highest ranked bean 300. However, if you examine CSPI's ranking of vegetables in the chapter

Glycemic Index of Grains

Grain	Glucose load
BREADS	
Barley kernel	34
Tortilla	38
Mixed grain	45
Oat bran	47
BREAKFAST CEREALS	
Rice Bran	19
All Bran	42
CEREAL GRAINS	
Barley	25
Rye rice	34
Wheat rice	41

Table adapted with permission from the *American Journal of Clinical Nutrition* 62 (1995): 871–935.

CSPI Food Value of Grains

Grain (5 oz. cooked)	Score
Quinoa	73
Macaroni or spaghetti, whole wheat	69
Amaranth	66
Buckwheat groats	64
Spaghetti, spinach	61
Bulgur	60
Barley, pearled	59
Wild rice	58
Millet	53
Brown rice	51
Triticale	47
Spaghetti	42
Wheat berries	41
Macaroni	39
Kamut	37
Oats, rolled	33
Spelt	33
White rice, converted	26
Couscous	23
White rice, instant	18
Soba noodles	12
Corn grits	10

CSPI came up with a score for each grain by adding its percent of the USRDA for five nutrients (magnesium, vitamin B_6, zinc, copper, and iron) plus fiber. There is no USRDA for fiber so they used the daily value of 25 grams in its place. Copyright 1993, CSPI. Reprinted and adapted from *Nutrition Action Healthletter* (1875 Connecticut Ave. N.W., Suite 300, Washington, D.C. 20009-5728; $24.00 for 10 issues).

"Hard Veggies" you'll see that high-ranking grains like quinoa outscore over twenty-eight different vegetables. Clearly the leading vegetables are a far more effective way of ingesting the most nutrients for the least number of calories. You will have to eat many more grains to achieve the same level of nutrition. However, many Americans find grains more attractive and easier to eat than veggies. If that's true of you, be certain to read the "Beans and Grains" chapter for an ideal way to get virtually all of your minerals and vitamins from non-vegetable sources. Since the grain most frequently used with beans is rice, let's take a minute to find the right kind. In the chart opposite you'll see that wild rice rates a score of 58, pretty decent, whereas instant white rice rates a measly 18. That white rice is not only nearly free of naturally occurring nutrients, its glucose load is 150 percent greater. CSPI nutritionist Bonnie Liebman says, "No matter where you buy wild rice, you'll pay a premium. It's rare and difficult to grow. But it's got more zinc than any other grain, and will give you a good dose of magnesium, fiber, and vitamin B_6 to boot. Don't be impressed by those commercial 'long grain and wild rice' mixtures. They're only about 10 percent wild rice."

Grains are an excellent source of the energy used for exercise. Where high animal fat meals have no positive effect on energy and leave many people feeling blah, a high-carbo meal, if you are active, increases your rate of breathing and metabolism, as if to point you toward your bike or stair machine. The greatest danger is for those sedentary individuals who carbo load like the pros. The biggest detriment for real athletes is carbo overloading on a daily basis instead of following hard workouts or in preparation for a race. Grains are also a good source of essential fatty acids.

SQUISHY

OK, these are the foods we were told to eat for a healthy lifestyle, but boy did someone sell us a bill of goods.

PASTA

Yep. The health food of the 1980s is heralded as the blood mud of the nineties. After a negative front-page story in the *New York Times,* pasta suffered a precipitous fall from grace in the American diet. In truth, that's slightly unfair. Pasta has a lower glucose load than many grain-based foods — far lower than rice. Here's where the problem lies. Since most pastas carry a medium glucose load, a diet high in pasta can quickly add up to a high total glucose load. The safest bet is small quantities of low glucose load, high-fiber pastas. Only whole wheat pastas have any fiber worth mentioning. They don't go down as fast as white flour pastas and may not taste as good, which means you'll eat a whole lot less pasta.

BREAD

Almost anything you buy in a supermarket is made with refined flours, then sprinkled with the whole grain *de jour,* so look at the label. Your best, safest bet are the mixed grain and oat bran breads that are low in sugar and high in fiber. From there on up, you'll find higher and higher glucose loads right up to the French baguette at 95, which might as well be a chocolate bar for all its health benefits. If you've been packing away breads in a move to eat healthy, you may find that this low-fiber content and high glucose load explain why you still can't get that belly fat to go away. With white flour and no fiber, there's little wonder that bagels beat out sugar.

BAKERY GOODS

You wouldn't expect much good news here, and there isn't. While muffins are at the lower end of the GI scale, many are still dripping with fat. A no-sugar, fat-free apple muffin is the best bet. Health food companies are making higher-fiber foods like these but be sure to look for products with less than 5 grams of sugar.

CRACKERS

They may say whole grain, but beware of how much of the white stuff is packed in. If it says wheat flour, stay away.

CEREAL GRAINS

Rice is the big surprise here, with white rice weighing in at 88, a glucose load higher than table sugar and most candy bars. That makes it little wonder that rice cakes, the diet food of choice for many low-fat junkies, can be the worst choice for protecting your glucose load with a stunning GI of 82. White rice, like white flour, is stripped of most minerals, vitamins, protein, and fiber. In fact, ½ cup of white rice has only 0.03 grams of dietary fiber. If you love rice, look for wild rice, which is high in fiber, B vitamins, calcium, phosphorus, Vitamin E, and iron. Leading experts call it "the food of the world."

Couscous, long assumed to be a low-load food, is also far higher than expected. Even if rice and couscous are eaten with super-low-glucose foods like soybeans, the combined glucose load climbs to the medium range.

CONVENIENCE FOODS

From potato chips and cupcakes to coffee cakes and fruit pies, these foods all carry a medium to high glucose load. The real danger is that they taste so darned good that you just can't stop. When loaded with corn syrup and hydrogenated oils, these have become the American waistline's public enemy number one.

Beans and Grains

Americans and Europeans are centerpiece diners. The centerpiece is the core of the meal, the glue binding it together, which sticks to our gut so we feel satisfied and full. When asked what we eat for lunch or dinner, most of us usually answer chicken, fish, steak, omelette — whatever the main protein course was is considered the centerpiece. That's our framework for describing a meal. The hardest part of getting Americans to accept a plant-based diet is that there doesn't appear to be a centerpiece. Eating a salad, some veggies, and beans just doesn't cut it. Ask the Annang in Nigeria what the meal's centerpiece is and they'll answer with whatever carbohydrate they've just eaten. The key to eating healthier plant-based meals is to get over the concept that meat has to be the centerpiece.

Conventional Wisdom
Meat is the centerpiece of any meal.

LEAN
Bean and grain combinations are the world's centerpiece.

ROAD MAP
You'll find the highest rated grain/bean combinations from the world's leading nutritional authorities. These are nearly perfect meals that fill you up, cut your hunger, and still provide nearly every nutrient required.

The best way to counter the centerpiece dilemma is to substitute another centerpiece. Since most Americans fear not eating enough protein at meals, it's important to know that the substitute does supply all the protein of the meat centerpiece. That's where bean/grain combinations come in. They provide complete proteins. But they go well beyond that to become a nearly perfect meal. They contain 48 of the 50 minerals and vitamins you require daily, plus the fiber necessary to bring down insulin, cholesterol, and blood glucose levels. In fact, the bean/grain combination far outweighs meats because if you eat *only* the bean/grain centerpiece you've had a complete healthy super meal. "If there's a magic bullet in foods it is the grain/bean combinations that are the magic meal," says Chris Kilham, author of the *Bread & Circus Whole Food Bible.* "All grains," says Chris, "go with beans. Some will taste better. It's a mix and match as you like approach. You get a complete meal from beans and grains. In combination grains and beans give you the profile that you need for all your protein."

BENEFITS

Complete meal: "Bean/grain combinations come pretty close to a complete meal. For one meal during the day, from a nutrient perspective, you will basically be fine. It comes quite close to meeting most of your nutritional requirements even if you never ate anything else. You would want to add a little vitamin C — an orange or anything citrus," says Harvard's Walter Willett. Martha Stone, professor of Food Science and Nutrition at Colorado State University, agrees. She says, "The grain and bean combination covers the amino acids that make it a complete protein, but you're missing vitamin C and you're also going to be missing iron, so you may want to add some raisins."

Weight control: Bean and grain combinations contain all of the weight control features listed in the "Hard Beans" chapter. Those range from the early and long-lasting satiety of soluble fibers to the energizing effects of tyrosine.

HARD COMBINATIONS

These are super-low-GI, high-soluble-fiber combinations.

LENTILS AND BARLEY

This is the number-one rated combination according to the University of Toronto's Dr. David Jenkins, inventor of the glucose load concept. "I would pick lentils and barley or oats. With lentils and barley, you'd have a complete meal. You've got lots of calcium. The only thing that might be missing of all the required nutrients is B_{12}. In the old days we picked B_{12} up out of the dirt and the earth that we ate with our food. Since we've become ultra clean and package things, we lack B_{12}. B_{12} is in low-fat cheeses and yogurts. It's found in plant products or fermented foods. You need some vitamin C as well. But this grain and bean combination should be eaten in the context of a good diet. If you prescribe this in isolation (without the backdrop of a good diet) you'll be open to a great deal of criticism."

HOMINY AND BLACK-EYE PEAS
SOYBURGER

This is a true, stick to your gut, fill you up fast, taste really terrific food which contains soy protein and a variety of grains and vegetables.

KASHA WITH NUTS AND BEANS

This is the favorite of Harvard's Dr. Walter Willet. "I usually have kasha for breakfast and have the leftovers with nuts, instead of beans, for lunch, which is exactly what you're proposing. If you want, you can add vitamin C from citrus or raisins for iron. The grain/bean combination is a good one."

Additional bean/grain combinations include:
- Garbanzos (chick peas) and millet
- Pink beans and whole wheat vermicelli
- Quinoa and pinto beans
- Brown rice and blackgraw dal (an Indian legume)
- Split peas or lentils with brown rice
- Wheat and oats with a combination of mung beans and split peas
- Mung beans and brown rice
- Lima beans and brown rice
- Wheat germ and split peas
- Kidney beans and whole wheat tortillas

CARBO BUSTER

If you're really dying for pasta now that it's made nutrition's triple XXX-rated list, consider eating pasta mixed with lentils or your favorite beans. The lentils really pull down the overall glucose load of the meal to make the pasta safe to eat. I first had this meal at the restaurant Mezzaluna in Aspen. The pasta makes the beans much more edible, while the beans keep your blood sugar in line. You can add olive oil to cut the GI load even further, but remember that one teaspoon contains 14 grams of fat. If you're at the time of day that you want the energizing effects of beans, by all means eat them alone. You don't have to eat the grain and bean simultaneously to get the complete protein. I'll have the beans, then wait thirty minutes or longer for the grain.

Try these combinations, then choose the two or three you like most to make as a snack or full-blown lunch or dinner. Most beans and grains complement each other so well that you just need to add spices or herbs for a great dish. The refreshing light feeling that comes over you after a grain/bean meal will quickly make them a favorite weapon in your arsenal.

SQUISHY

It's hard to believe you can ruin such a made-in-heaven combination, but, by God, food processors have managed. As an example, look at the instant bean and rice dishes found in many supermarkets and health food stores. If they've shaved or pummelled the beans into tiny little pieces, all you need to do is add water to make them into perfect mush. They are no longer hard. Combine that with the sky-high GI of rice and you might as well have had a jelly sandwich with a little added fiber. Fast-food bean tacos are another example where the combination of refried beans, cheese, sour cream, and a white flour taco will make you wonder what hit you.

Hard Veggies

The world's healthiest diets from Asian to Cretan are considered largely vegetarian. Even our meat-eating prehistoric ancestors complemented their kills only with vegetables. You too can make veggies as big a part of your diet as you like. If you're not a veggie fan or if you're sick to death of limp, wasted restaurant and company cafeteria vegetables, at the end of this chapter I've included two intriguing ways to get your veggies.

Conventional Wisdom
Bulk up with carbos.

LEAN
Bulk with veggies.

ROAD MAP

This chapter has lists for hunger-cutting veggies, veggies that cut your blood sugar, the most filling veggies, and the most nutritious ones. First choose vegetables to kill your hunger, then those that cut your blood sugar level. Then look for high-bulk veggies as fillers and high-nutrient veggies to balance your diet.

VEGETABLES THAT CONTROL YOUR WEIGHT
HUNGER-CUTTING VEGETABLES
High-Soluble-Fiber Veggies

The high-soluble-fiber values here are potent medicine for tempering any rise in blood sugar. Because these vegetables have extremely few calories, you can eat all you want. The more the better.

Soluble Fiber in Vegetables

Vegetable	Soluble fiber (per 400 calories)
Brussels sprouts, fresh	3
Okra pods, fresh, trimmed	2.9
Parsley, fresh	2.8
Brussels sprouts, cooked	2.5
Celeriac, fresh	2.4
Parsnip, cooked	2.3
Turnip, cooked	2.2
Cabbage, winter savoy, fresh	2

Table adapted with permission from HCF Nutrition Research, Inc.

Low Glucose Load Vegetables

OK, so I goofed. I could only find one veggie, the dried pea, that cuts your blood sugar. There's little surprise that veggies can have a high glucose load. They are meant to entice you to eat them for their storehouse of minerals and vitamins. The real villains here are plain potatoes, which have a strikingly high glucose load. While the sweet potato still has a moderate glucose load, you'll see that it's a high-rated vegetable for its storehouse of nutrients. For that one time during the day when you really need a carbo boost fast, grab a sweet potato. French fries enter onto the triple XXX-rated list for having a high glucose load added to a sky-high fat content. High-load veggies should be paired with low-GI foods to blunt their impact.

Low Glucose Load Vegetables

Vegetable	Glucose Load
Peas, dried	22
Green peas	48
Yam	51
Sweet potato	54
Sweet corn	55
Pontiac, boiled	56
White potato	56
Avon, canned	61
New potato	62
Prince Edward Island, boiled	63
Beetroot	64
White mashed potato	70

Low Glucose Load Vegetables

Vegetable	Glucose Load
Carrots	71
Swede	72
Potato, boiled, mashed	73
French fries	75
Pumpkin	75
Potato, instant	83
Potato, baked	85
Parsnips	97

Table adapted with permission from the *American Journal of Clinical Nutrition* 62 (1995): 871–935.

MOST FILLING VEGETABLES: HIGH BULK   Vegetables are the premier food for getting the maximum amount of food bulk for the minimum number of calories. You could literally eat all you want with little fear of gaining weight. Grains give you bulk, but they carry lots of extra calories by comparison. Large amounts of high-bulk veggies require a substantial amount of energy to digest, which can increase your metabolism. According to Luke Bucci, Ph.D., one in particular, hot chili peppers, can increase the number of calories you burn at rest. Through his research he discovered that you can raise your metabolic rate by about 2 to 5 percent for about 3 hours.

In the table below, the number opposite each vegetable is the number of pounds you would have to eat to ingest 2,500 calories.

You'll also see lettuce ranks incredibly high in bulk, but remember that you'd have to eat nearly forty pounds a day to hit 2,500 calories. If you do bulk up on lettuce, just leave the dressing behind.

High-Bulk Vegetables

Vegetable	Bulk (pounds per 2,500 calories)
Cabbage, Chinese	39
Lettuce	39
Celery	32.8
Cucumber	32.8
Radish	32.1
Zucchini	32.1
Eggplant	28.8
Squash	28.8
Endive	27.3
Peppers, chili	27.3
Tomato	27.3
Watercress	27.3
Artichoke	26
Cabbage	22.8
Beans, green	21.9
Asparagus	21
Spinach	21
Bamboo shoots	20.2
Cauliflower	20.2

High-Bulk Vegetables

Vegetable	Bulk (pounds per 2,500 calories)
Mushrooms	19.5
Turnip	19.5
Mustard greens	17.6
Broccoli	17.1
Beans, mung sprout	15.6
Okra	15.2
Onion, green	15.2
Onion	14.8
Lychee	14
Carrot	13
Seaweed (konbu)	12.7
Beets	12.7
Brussels sprouts	12.1
Collards	12.1
Seaweed (wakame)	12.1
Ginger	11.9
Kale	10.3
Poi	9.11

MOST NUTRITIOUS VEGETABLES Vegetables are the single densest source of minerals and vitamins. You're getting the greatest number of nutrients for the fewest number of calories. Look at the scores in the following list and you will see that they are off the charts, ranking higher than all other food groups. Collard greens at 461 is the king of all foods for nutrient content.

CSPI Food Value of Vegetables

Vegetable (⅓ cup unless other quantity given)	Score
Collard greens, frozen	461
Spinach	424
Kale	410
Swiss chard	322
Red pepper, raw, ½	309
Sweet potato, no skin	285
Pumpkin, canned	252
Carrots	241
Broccoli	179
Carrot, raw, 1	171
Okra	165
Brussels sprouts	143
Lettuce, 1 cup shredded	141
Potato, baked, with skin	136
Spinach, raw, 1 cup	130
Squash, winter	129
Green pepper, raw, ½	112
Mixed vegetables, frozen	112
Parsley, raw	97
Broccoli, raw, ½ cup	91
Snow peas, frozen	89
Peas, frozen	88
Asparagus	84
Endive, raw, 1 cup chopped	82
Tomato, raw, ½	76
Avocado, California, raw	71
Artichoke, ½	68
Potato, baked, no skin	67
Cauliflower	64
Lettuce, Boston or bibb	59
Cauliflower, raw, ½ cup	58
Squash, summer	56
Green beans	54

CSPI Food Value of Vegetables

Vegetable (⅓ cup unless other quantity given)	Score
Parsnip	54
Celery, raw, ½ cup	50
Corn	50
Rutabaga	50
Cabbage	44
Cabbage, red, raw, ½	43
Green beans, canned	42
Lettuce, iceberg, 1 cup	40
Corn, frozen	38
Beets, canned, ½ cup	32
Mushrooms	32
Onions	31
Turnips	30
Radishes, raw, ¼ cup	18
Cucumber, raw, ½ cup	14
Onions, raw, ¼ cup	14
Eggplant	13
Mushrooms, raw, ½ cup	12
Alfalfa sprouts, raw, ½ cup	7
Garlic, raw, 1 clove	3

CSPI came up with a score for each vegetable by adding up its percent of the Daily Value for five nutrients (vitamin C, folate, potassium, calcium, and iron) plus carotenoids and fiber. There is no Daily Value for carotenoids, so they made up their own, 5,000 micrograms. Copyright 1996, CSPI. Reprinted and adapted from *Nutrition Action Healthletter* (1875 Connecticut Ave. N.W., Suite 300, Washington, D.C. 20009-5728; $24.00 for 10 issues).

The sad truth is that vegetables that fall off the end of the list can be a waste of time to eat. They contain vanishingly few nutrients, and when added to salad or dressings are far worse than eating nothing at all. In an article in *Nutrition Action,* Bonnie Liebman writes, "Many of America's favorite vegetables — like iceberg lettuce and celery — are among the least nutritious. The typical salad, for example, combines some of the least nutritious vegetables. Its base is iceberg lettuce, now the second most popular American vegetable after potatoes. Eat a whole cup of iceberg and you get ten percent of the USRDA for nothing! Likewise for salad vegetables like cucumbers, alfalfa sprouts, and raw mushrooms. Only tomatoes exceed 10 percent of the USRDA for vitamin C — if you eat half a tomato." Spinach or romaine lettuce is a much better pick, says Bonnie.

HOW TO EAT YOUR VEGGIES
MEDITERRANEAN STYLE

If you're really down on eating limp, mushy vegetables, here's a great no-compromise solution. This is the heart of the Mediterranean diet. They are vegetables sautéed in olive oil. This goes a long way to satisfying your fat craving and can be a great deal healthier than a big dousing of low-fat but high-sugar salad dressings. This is a highly satisfying way of cutting your glycemic load and slowing down stomach emptying for longer satiety. If you're not a huge olive oil fan, you can mix in canola oil instead. Just be certain it's not hydrogenated.

THE VITA-MIXER

This was the most popular item in my last book, *Turning Back the Clock.* The Vita-Mixer crushes a plateful of veggies and fruits so you can drink them in one simple serving. This is an easy task to perform when you come home in the evening, and it is a great way to bulk up. The veggies do lose their hardness, which increases their GI, but that's the price you pay for ease of preparation. The device is recommended by the Center for Science in the Public Interest in Washington, D.C. The Vita-Mixer has a 37,000 rpm, nearly two-horsepower lawn-mower-quality engine that can blast pulp, fiber, even seeds into smithereens. Standard juicers leave juice so gritty you may find them unpleasant to drink. The Vita-Mixer produces a smooth puree. The manufacturer claims that all the nutrients are retained and that the machine liberates more of them than even our own digestive systems could. There are two recipes in the "Feedforward Eating" chapter of the book.

Hard Fruits

Fruits are largely overrated food for dieters because of the "all fruits are equal" axiom. Pick the wrong fruits, fruit juices, or fruit-laced foods, and you'll add pounds. Pick the right fruits and you'll hit upon a treasure trove of foods with all the key ingredients for success from high soluble fiber and bulk to a low glucose load.

Conventional Wisdom
Fruits are a dieter's delight.

LEAN
Pick your fruits with care.

ROAD MAP
This chapter has lists for hunger-cutting fruits, fruits that cut your blood sugar, the most filling fruits, and fruits with the most nutrients. First choose hunger-cutting fruits, then fruits that cut your blood sugar. Then look for high-bulk fruits as fillers and high-nutrient fruits to balance your diet. The end of the chapter deals with squishy fruits, which have the most potential to make you fat.

HUNGER-CUTTING FRUITS (HIGH SOLUBLE FIBER)
Only dried fruits have a high amount of soluble fiber, with apricots leading the way. By combining fruits with oat bran, food manufacturers attain a higher level of soluble fiber.

Be sure to look out for concentrated sugars in dried fruits. A cup of apricots has 50 grams of sugar, peaches 71 grams, and that's without any added sugars. "If you're watching your calories, you should

Soluble Fiber in Fruits

Fruit and Fruit-based Products	Soluble Fiber (per 100 g.)
Apricots, dried	4.4
Figs, dried	4
Peaches, dried	3.8
Prunes, dried	3.8
Oat Bran Fancy Fruit Muffin	2.4
Oat Bran Fruit Jumbo Cookies	2.4
Oat Bran raisin muffin	2.1
Oat Bran Fruit and Nut Cookies	2
Oat Bran Jumbo Fruit Bar	2

Table adapted with permission from HCF Nutrition Research Foundation, Inc.

watch your intake of dried fruit," advises Elsie Cunningham of the American Dietetic Association.

LOW GLUCOSE LOAD FRUITS

These fruits have a low glucose load. They are ranked from the lowest load fruits, cherries.

Look at the tables above and below and you'll see that apricots are a surprise winner with a high amount of soluble fiber.

Glycemic Index of Fruits

Cherries	22
Plum	24
Grapefruit	25
Peach, fresh	28
Peach, canned, natural juice	30

Glycemic Index of Fruits

Apricots, dried	31
Apple	36
Pear	36

Table adapted with permission from the *American Journal of Clinical Nutrition* 62 (1995): 871–935.

HIGH-BULK FRUITS; MOST-FILLING FRUITS

Any of the top-ranking fruits provides a great way to add lots of bulk to keep you full. However, since most fruits are relatively low in fiber, you won't notice the same satiety that you get with beans or high-fiber breakfast cereals, leading to that full but empty feeling, so don't rely on fruits alone to keep you full. The world's healthiest diets do

High-Bulk Fruits

Fruit	Bulk
Lemon	30.4
Grapefruit	27.3
Kumquat	22.8
Watermelon	21
Cantaloupe	18.2
Melon	18.2
Peach	16.6
Pumpkin	16.6
Tangerine	16.1
Orange	15.6
Loquat	14.8
Strawberries	14.8
Cranberries	12.4
Grapes	11.9
Apricot	11.4

High-Bulk Fruits

Fruit	Bulk
Pineapple	10.5
Apple	9.42
Blackberries	9.42
Nectarine	9.26
Plum	9.11
Pear	8.96
Blueberries	8.81
Loganberries	8.81
Cherries	8.67
Mango	8.28
Raspberries	7.48
Fig	6.83
Prune	6.83
Banana	6.43
Raisins	3.64

both, combining huge amounts of bulky fruit with high bean and vegetable content. The table above ranks bulk for fruits, with the highest ranked first. The value correlates with the number of pounds of the fruit you would have to ingest to consume 2,500 calories.

Wonder why some bright guy got the idea for a grapefruit diet? Look at how it scores in this table. You see that you would have to eat 27 pounds of grapefruit to reach an intake of 2,500 calories. That made the grapefruit diet possible. You just couldn't get 27 pounds of grapefruit into you no matter how much you ate.

While the grapefruit diet isn't recommended, a diet high in a variety of these foods will provide lots of weight-losing bulk: Note that raisins and bananas at the bottom end are low bulk and high glucose load . . . not much use for weight control.

MOST NUTRITIOUS FRUITS

Here's how fruit ranks for minerals, vitamins, and fiber. The top of the list, papaya, beats all but two fruits for its nutrient content. Either papaya or cantaloupe provides almost a complete daily dose of vitamins A and C, with a hefty helping of potassium. Cantaloupe, though, is the best bet overall since it provides high bulk with sky-

Fruit	Score	Fruit	Score
Papaya (½)	252	Apple, with skin (1)	58
Cantaloupe (¼)	213	Boysenberries (1 cup)	57
Strawberries (1 cup)	186	Pears (1)	48
Oranges (1)	169	Grapes, green (60)	46
Tangerines (2)	168	Peaches, canned in juice	43
Kiwi (1)	154	Apple, no skin (1)	42
Mango (½)	153	Pineapple, canned in juice	40
Apricots (4)	143	Figs, dried (2)	39
Persimmons (1)	134	Currants, dried (¼ cup)	36
Watermelon (2 cups)	122	Rhubarb, cooked (½ cup)	36
Raspberries (1 cup)	117	Raisins (¼ cup, packed)	35
Grapefruit, red or pink (½)	103	Dates (5)	30
Blackberries (1 cup)	101	Pears, canned in juice	16
Apricots, dried (10)	97		
Grapefruit, white (½)	84		
Honeydew melon (⅒)	81		
Peaches (2)	77		
Pineapple (1 cup)	77		
Star fruit (1)	73		
Blueberries (1 cup)	68		
Cherries, sweet (1 cup)	64		
Nectarine (1)	64		
Pomegranate (1)	61		
Banana (1)	60		
Plums (2)	60		
Prunes, dried (5)	59		

CSPI came up with a score for each fruit by adding its percent of the USRDA for nine nutrients (vitamin A, vitamin C, potassium, folate, niacin, thiamin, iron, riboflavin, and calcium) plus fiber. There are no USRDA's for fiber or potassium so they used the Daily Value of 25 grams for fiber and their own RDA of 3,500 milligrams for potassium. Copyright 1992, CSPI. Reprinted and adapted from *Nutrition Action Healthletter* (1875 Connecticut Ave. N.W., Suite 300, Washington, D.C. 20009-5728; $24.00 for 10 issues).

high nutrients. Notice, however, how many lower-ranking fruits, such as raisins, rhubarb, and apples, are also higher in calories.

Does an apple a day keep the doctor away? You stand a much better shot at staying beyond his clutches with over a dozen other fruits, from strawberries to kiwis and apricots. By choosing high-ranking, low-calorie items, you can make fruits work to peel off the pounds. But they must be hard fruits.

SQUISHY: FRUIT'S DARK SIDE

When sugar junkies wean themselves off refined flours and sugars, some turn to fruit for a replacement. Because the sugar in fruit, which is fructose, doesn't light up the glucose receptors in the brain, dieters don't get the glucose/endorphin rush. In an ill-fated attempt to experience that rush, the sugar lover will overeat fruits with high amounts of fructose, such as bananas, raisins, prunes, and figs.

While dieters are often encouraged to splurge on juices and fruits, those items can also make you fat. When large amounts of fructose are ingested, they can increase the production of fat in your liver, with more ending up in your blood vessel walls and around your waist.

High-sugar fruits canned in syrup have at least a medium glucose load, but the worst are fruit juices. Juices are to fruit what white flour is to whole grain. That's why it's best to stick with fresh fruits that have a low glucose index or that have high amounts of fiber, which can act to fill you up and blunt your blood sugar. Along with refined carbos, high-GI fruits are the two most common reasons dieters don't lose the last five pounds of ring-around-the-middle body fat.

You wouldn't expect to find a high glucose load for fruits and yet many of them are out of the park, like watermelon, pineapple, and rockmelon. For comparison's sake, consider real sugars. Fructose weighs in with a rock bottom 23. Table sugar or sucrose registers 65.

This table shows fruits starting with medium and ending with high glucose loads.

"FRUIT-JUICE SWEETENED"

Fruit sweeteners are boiled-down fruit. Manufacturers boil it down until there's only sugar. What you get is a combination of glucose, fructose, and sucrose. It's a syrup that's referred to as "concentrate." These products may be labeled "no sugar." But let's take a closer look. Fruit-juice-sweetened food is little different from foods that use white sugar or corn syrup, claims the Center for Science in the Public Interest. These juices are usually stripped of flavor and color. They have only tiny amounts of vitamins or minerals. Stripped juices are little more than sugar water. If you look at the first ingredient on peach fruit juice, you find that it's grape juice concentrate. In *Nutrition Action Healthletter,* Jim Tillotson, director of the Food Policy Institute at Tufts University, gave this advice: "In the supermarket, if I

Glucose Load in Fruits

Fruit	Glucose Load
Grapes	43
Orange	43
Pineapple juice	46
Grapefruit juice	48
Kiwi	52
Peach, canned, light syrup	52
Banana	53
Fruit cocktail, canned	55
Mango	55
Sultanas	56
Orange juice	57
Peach, canned, heavy syrup	58
Raisins	64
Pineapple	66
Watermelon	72
Rockmelon	95

Table adapted with permission from the *American Journal of Clinical Nutrition* 62 (1995): 871–935.

saw white grape, apple, or pear juice concentrate, I'd be suspicious." According to nutrition scientist Luke Bucci, Ph.D., of Weider Nutrition in Salt Lake City, Utah, fruit sweeteners are not any better than table sugar. Many health food products use fruit juice sweeteners to make them appear healthy.

"MADE WITH REAL FRUIT"

Great claim, but how much real fruit? In convenience stores and supermarkets this label requires close scrutiny. Many fruit juice manufacturers use white grape juice sweeteners, grape juice concentrate, and other stripped sugars as their main source of "fruit." The real fruit they have is in near trace amounts. One children's snack has one-seventeenth of an orange. Another company's cereal bar has one-fiftieth of an apple.

15

Hard Fast Foods

Convenience has become the driving force behind food selection for on-the-go Americans. Nowhere does adherence to a great weight-control program go south faster than on the road. Tepary beans and mesquite soup give way to limp, fat-soaked airline pasta. Hummus and whole wheat are replaced by lunch counter burgers and fries. Market research shows that consumers make the unfortunate error of failing to think about food until hunger strikes, then reach out and grab the quickest, easiest item to eat. Whole food pioneer Jim Rosen, president of Fantastic Foods in Petaluma, California, observes, "The problem is that the foods you can grab the fastest are the least nutritious — a candy bar, something out of a vending machine, a bag of chips, a burger from McDonald's." The unavailability of food is what kept our ancestors thin. The hunt was the thing. Now the hunt is no farther than a dollar bill that's smooth enough to slide into a vending machine without being rejected.

Conventional Wisdom
They've got to be fast.

LEAN
They've got to be hard and fast.

ROAD MAP

There is a great misapprehension that there is just too much time and effort involved in foraging for great foods . . . that you have to spend hours over the stove in the evenings preparing beans and oatmeal for the next day. This chapter brings you great fast foods and snack foods. You needn't buy many of them. Find ones you like, then stock up on ample quantities to take with you to the office, school, and on the road. The chapter has both off-the-shelf fast foods and do-it-yourself weight-control champs.

VARIETIES OF HARD FAST FOODS

Hard fast foods come in several varieties which include dehydrated foods, food bars, packaged foods, and picnic style. Here's a look.

BOIL 'EM AND SOAK 'EM: DEHYDRATED FOODS

These are dehydrated dishes that are reconstituted by adding boiling water. They're analogous to dried fruit. Since water gives bacteria the medium in which to grow, you can transport them when they are dehydrated. Future technologies will allow some moisture to be left in these dishes so they can be eaten without adding boiling water. This is one of the very best ways of providing portable whole foods. The downsides are the added sodium and the degree to which the processing shreds or tears the foods. I have a hot water heater at the office that takes less than sixty seconds to boil enough water to reconstitute one of these dehydrated dishes. They're incredibly cheap. At less than $2.00 you have a complete small meal or snack. These are great retaliation for bad airline food. When the flight attendant asks: "Chicken or beef?" You reply: "Hot water, please." You'll have a much better and healthier meal.

SOUPS

Nile Spice Black Bean Soup
Ingredients: Black beans, dehydrated vegetables (tomatoes, onions, red peppers), garlic, salt, spices, brown rice syrup powder, yeast extract.

Calories: 170	Carbohydrates: 35 grams
Fat: 1.5 grams	Fiber: 11 grams
Saturated Fat: 0	Sugars: 3 grams
Cholesterol: 0	Protein: 11 grams
Sodium: 600 mg	

Fantastic Foods Five Bean Soup

Ingredients: Precooked pinto, black, pink, red, and white beans, de-hydrated potatoes, tomatoes, onions, carrots, garlic, celery, beets, pre-cooked lentils, brown rice syrup powder, dried yeast, miso powder (soybeans, rice, salt), salt, yeast extract, natural smoke flavor, spices.

Serving size: 1 packet	Sodium: 480 mg
Calories: 230	Carbohydrates: 43 grams
Fat: 1 gram	Fiber: 10 grams ★★★★
Saturated fat: 0	Sugars: 4 grams
Cholesterol: 0	Protein: 12 grams

Fantastic Foods is one of America's best-known companies for portable health foods. They produce over sixty instant, all-natural vegetarian meals and side dishes. Their slogan is "Healthy Meals for a Hectic World," i.e., you can take it with you.

In addition to their soups, which are filled with dehydrated ingredients, Fantastic Foods has just come out with a line of instant organic cereals. The hot cereals include: cinnamon apple tamale; banana nut barley with millet; whole wheat with blueberries, strawberries and raspberries; and cranberry, orange tamale.

Fantastic Foods has become the prototype of portable health food. I use some of their foods on the road and applaud what they do. However, some products are compromised by the degree the ingredients are refined into a smaller particle size and by the requirement for boiled water. Both of these increase glucose load and the rate of food absorption.

Rather than buy the whole line, choose those items which have high fiber without much added salt or sugar. These products are manufactured by companies that believe in the quality of whole foods, offering people high-fiber or high-protein nutritious real food. Even the worst of them is far better than any fast food on the market. They beat the pants off vending machine and airline fare.

Taste Adventures Five Bean Chili

Take a look at the amount of protein in Taste Adventures Five Bean Chili — 19 grams! Ray Williams, who along with his wife, Ann, founded this Harbor City, California–based company, tells me that the idea for this soup came from a customer who combined their black bean, red bean, and lentil soups, submitted the concoction for a chili cook-off contest, and won! All you have to do is add water, stir, and eat.

Ingredients: Precooked beans (red beans, black beans, white beans, lentils, pinto beans), textured soy flour, tomatoes, mild chili peppers, herbs and spices, bell peppers, onions, sea salt, garlic, and citric acid.

Serving size: ¾ cup	Sodium: 490 mg
Calories: 240	Carbohydrates: 45 grams
Fat: 1.5 grams	Fiber: 14 grams
Saturated fat: 0	Sugars: 8 grams
Cholesterol: 0	Protein: 19 grams

CEREALS

*** *Fantastic Foods Banana Nut Barley*
Ingredients: Organic precooked rolled whole barley, crystallized cane juice, organic cracked barley, pecans, dried bananas, sea salt, natural flavors.

Serving size: 1 package	Sodium: 230 mg
Calories: 180	Carbohydrates: 35 grams
Fat: 2.5 grams	Fiber: 4 grams
Saturated fat: 0	Sugars: 7 grams
Cholesterol: 0	Protein: 4 grams

This one breakfast cereal has a little less fiber and a little more sugar than I'd like, but it's one of the few games in town when it comes to a totally portable hot breakfast cereal.

Kashi Pilaf
Ingredients: Whole oats, long-grain brown rice, whole rye, whole hard red winter wheat, whole triticale, whole buckwheat, whole barley, sesame seeds.

Serving size: ½ cup	Sodium: 15 mg
Calories: 170	Carbohydrates: 30 grams
Fat: 3 grams	Fiber: 6 grams
Saturated fat: 0	Sugars: 0
Cholesterol: 0	Protein: 6 grams

MIX AND MATCH

The first key of a hard fast food is portability. Margaret Wittenberg, author of *Good Food* and Whole Foods Market's Food and Nutrition research director, says, "When you talk about portability, it's like going on a picnic." The mix-and-match approach is best applied to grains and beans. Since there is almost no good totally portable single product, like a meal bar, you end up combining ingredients on the road. Carry them as separate components and then mix them in the field. The beauty of this approach is that you only need two components, beans and grains, to give you a nutritionally complete meal that supplies 95 percent of all your minerals and vitamins.

Mixing and matching can be tough for novices. So, I asked Margaret to help out with some suggestions free of artificial sweeteners, colors, flavors, and preservatives, added growth hormones, antibiotics, nitrates, or other chemicals or bleached or bromated grain products. At the top of her list are grain/bean combinations. "The grocery industry understands the value of beans and is trying to offer them to the public through soups or dips, in jars or containers, or hummus." (She often brings bean dips and crackers on trips.) The combination of the bean dips and grain crackers or breads gives you complete proteins and nearly all your micronutrients. Crackers and bean paste make an even faster combination. Pick up great whole grain crackers, bread, or corn tortillas and a jar of bean paste plus a knife. You can make a complete meal out of it anywhere you go. I tried this first at a hotel in Austin, Texas, instead of a Snickers bar. I felt a tremendous sense of calm come over me and had the best night's sleep I can remember. By mixing bean paste with a really high-quality cracker, you've got the perfect meal: nearly all your micronutrients plus complete proteins and slow-burning carbos. This is a great substitute for cheese and crackers.

Santa Cruz MediterrAsian Dip (Hummus with Wasabi) and Lieken Urkorn Graham Wholemeal Wheat Bread
Ingredients: Garbanzo beans, sesame tahini, water, lemon juice, red bell pepper, white vinegar, lime juice, wasabi (horseradish), olive oil, sesame oil, sea salt, garlic, natural spices.

Serving size: 2 Tbsp.   Sodium: 109 mg
Calories: 75   Carbohydrates: 10.2 grams
Fat: 2.7 grams   Fiber: 2.7 grams
Saturated fat: 0   Sugars: 0
Cholesterol: 0   Protein: 3.3 grams

Ingredients: Wholemeal wheat flour, natural leaven made from group rye, salt, yeast.

Serving size: 1 slice   Sodium: 230 mg
Calories: 130   Carbohydrates: 26 grams
Fat: 1.5 grams   Fiber: 4 grams
Saturated fat: 0   Sugars: 1 gram
Cholesterol: 0   Protein: 4 grams

Garden of Eatin' Spicy Chipotle Red Bean Dip and Lieken Urkorn Sunflower Whole Kernel Rye Bread

Ingredients: Organic red beans, organic tomatoes, organic onions, organic apple cider vinegar, chipotle chiles, lime juice, salt, cumin, organic cilantro, coriander, oregano, organic jalapeño chiles.

Serving size: 2 Tbsp.   Sodium: 90 mg
Calories: 25   Carbohydrates: 5 grams
Fat: 0   Fiber: 2 grams
Saturated fat: 0   Sugars: less than 1 gram
Cholesterol: 0   Protein: 1 gram

Ingredients: Ground rye, natural leaven, water, wholemeal wheat flour, sunflower seeds, barley, salt, yeast

Serving size: 1 slice   Sodium: 290 mg
Calories: 150   Carbohydrates: 29 grams
Fat: 2 grams   Fiber: 5 grams
Saturated fat: 0   Sugars: 3 grams
Cholesterol: 0   Protein: 5 grams

Casbah Instant Hummus (Garbanzo Dip) and Wasa Multi Grain Crisp Bread

Ingredients: Garbanzo beans, sesame tahini, garlic, natural lemon powder, salt, spices.

Serving size: 1 oz.   Saturated fat: 0
Calories: 160   Cholesterol: 0
Fat: 8 grams   Sodium: 180 mg

Carbohydrates: 14 grams	Sugars: 0
Fiber: 1 gram	Protein: 5 grams

Ingredients: Whole grain rye flour, oat flakes, whole grain wheat flour, barley flour, whole grain oat flour, yeast, mono and diglycerides, salt.

Serving size: 1 slice	Sodium: 85 mg
Calories: 45	Carbohydrates: 8 grams
Fat: 0	Fiber: 2 grams
Saturated fat: 0	Sugars: 0
Cholesterol: 0	Protein: 2 grams

Health Valley Mild or Spicy Vegetarian Chili with Lentils and Kavli Whole Grain Rye Crispbread

Ingredients: Water, organic tomatoes, organic lentils, onions, organic tomato paste, soy granules, organic carrots, honey, sea salt, garlic powder, chili pepper, cumin, paprika, cayenne pepper, organic sage, organic basil, oregano.

Serving size: ½ cup	Sodium: 100 mg
Calories: 80	Carbohydrates: 14 grams
Fat: 0	Fiber: 6 grams
Saturated fat: 0	Sugars: 3 grams
Cholesterol: 0	Protein: 7 grams

Ingredients: Whole rye flour, whole wheat flour, water and salt.

Serving size: 2 pieces	Sodium: 55 mg
Calories: 70	Carbohydrates: 15 grams
Fat: 0.5 grams	Fiber: 3 grams
Saturated fat: 0	Sugars: 0
Cholesterol: 0	Protein: 2 grams

Bearitos Beans & Rice Cuban Style and Alvarado Street Sprouted Wheat Tortillas

Ingredients: Water, organic black beans (soaked in water), onion, bell peppers, carrots, tomatoes, brown rice, tomato paste, whole wheat flour, spices, potato starch, sea salt, garlic powder.

Serving size: 1 cup	Saturated fat: 0
Calories: 150	Cholesterol: 0
Fat: 1 gram	Sodium: 490 mg

Carbohydrates: 27 grams   Sugars: 2 grams
Fiber: 5 grams   Protein: 7 grams
Ingredients: Organic whole wheat berries, organic whole wheat flour, water, unrefined safflower oil, sea salt, baking powder.

Serving size: 1 tortilla   Sodium: 250 mg
Calories: 130   Carbohydrates: 26 grams
Fat: 1 gram   Fiber: 1 gram
Saturated fat: 0   Sugars: 12 grams
Cholesterol: 0   Protein: 4 grams

Guiltless Gourmet Mild Black Bean Dip and Guiltless Gourmet Unsalted Tortilla Chips

Ingredients: Water, black beans, distilled vinegar, bell peppers, apple cider vinegar, jalapeño peppers, spices, onion powder, salt, garlic, beet powder, citric acid, dried torula yeast.

Serving size: 2 Tbsp.   Sodium: 100 mg
Calories: 30   Carbohydrates: 5 grams
Fat: 0   Fiber: 1 gram
Saturated fat: 0   Sugars: 1 gram
Cholesterol: 0   Protein: 2 grams

Ingredients: Yellow corn, lime.

Serving size: 20 chips   Sodium: 26 mg
Calories: 110   Carbohydrates: 22 grams
Fat: 1 gram   Fiber: 2 grams
Saturated fat: 0   Sugars: less than 1 gram
Cholesterol: 0   Protein: 2 grams

Here are some additional snacks I like that you can include as part of any combination:

Ak-Mak 100% Whole Wheat Stone Ground Sesame Crackers

Ingredients: Stone ground whole wheat flour, water, clover honey, sesame oil, dairy butter, sesame seeds, yeast, salt.

Serving size: 5 crackers   Sodium: 213.55 mg
Calories: 116   Carbohydrates: 19 grams
Fat: 2.27 grams   Fiber: 3.5 grams
Saturated fat: 0.48 grams   Sugars: 2.28 grams
Cholesterol: 0   Protein: 4.61 grams

Mestemacher All-Natural Famous German Fitness Bread
Ingredients: Rye kernels, water, whole rye flour, oat kernels, whole
wheat flour, wheat germ, sea salt, yeast.

Serving size: 1 slice	Sodium: 340 mg
Calories: 110	Carbohydrates: 20 grams
Fat: 1 gram	Fiber: 6 grams
Saturated fat: 1 gram	Sugars: 0
Cholesterol: 0	Protein: 4 grams

BARS

Most bars are still at a very primitive stage as a hard fast food. Since
most technologies rely on extrusion, most have some kind of a sugar
base. The sugar may be a fruit-juice mix, maltodextrin, rice syrup, or
corn syrup, all of which are pretty trashy forms of carbohydrate.
Some advanced bars add grains. But the ultimate, meal-in-a-bar combination of grains and beans has yet to see the light of day. I'd be one
of the first people to buy a grain/bean bar. Make sure the bar you
choose doesn't list some kind of syrup or other goo as its first ingredient. If you choose carefully you can buy bars that have a very low
glucose load. Here are some of the better ones. Zbar leads the list of
well-designed, low-GI bars, although it is low in fiber.

Zbar
Ingredients: Cornstarch, sorbitol, soy protein isolate, maltitol syrup,
crisp rice (rice flour, malt extract, rice bran), polydextrose, cocoa
(processed with alkali), nonfat milk, glycerine, canola oil, natural flavors, arabic gum, lecithin.

Serving size: 1 bar	Sodium: 95 mg
Calories: 110	Carbohydrates: 22 grams
Fat: 2.5 grams	Fiber: less than 1 gram
Saturated fat: 0	Sugars: 2 grams
Cholesterol: 0	Protein: 5 grams

Zbar is engineered food with proven medicinal properties. It leads the
way for industry to create fast foods for health. Although the Zbar is
intended for people with diabetes, it can be used by anybody wanting
to regulate and stabilize blood glucose levels.

The Zbar is made with uncooked cornstarch because it has a very low glycemic index and is very slowly absorbed in the gut.

The manufacturer, Baker Norton, plans to study whether this bar can control appetite. Says Lisa Raskin Mervis, M.S., R.D., C.D.E., a company advisory board member, "We know intuitively that it should help to prevent hunger over a long period of time. We believe this because (a) it doesn't have so much sugar that it will cause a spike in your insulin secretion and (b) it absorbs at such a slow rate it will keep you from getting hungry."

You can find Zbar, which costs 99 cents per bar and comes in boxes of five bars, in pharmacies.

The remaining bars have much higher amounts of sugar.

**Extreme Energy Nutrition Bar

Ingredients: Oat flour, honey, rice syrup, whole wheat flour, defatted wheat germ, roasted buckwheat, rolled oats, almonds, peanuts, natural flavors.

Serving size: 1 bar	Sodium: 65 mg
Calories: 230	Carbohydrates: 44 grams
Fat: 3 grams	Fiber: 5 grams
Saturated fat: 0.5 gram	Sugars: 20 grams
Cholesterol: 0	Protein: 7 grams

Gary Null's Fiber & Fruit Bar

Ingredients: Natural assorted fruits (raisins, apples, and/or prunes), rice bran fiber, honey, unsweetened carob flour, unsweetened carbo coating, natural flavors, choline, inositol, L-Carnitine, buchu leaves.

Serving size: 1 bar	Sodium: 32 mg
Calories: 155	Carbohydrates: 27 grams
Fat: less than 3 grams	Fiber: 6 grams
Saturated fat: 0	Sugars: 13 grams
Cholesterol: 0	Protein: 5 grams

Clif Bar

Ingredients: Rolled oats, FruitSource sweetener (whole rice syrup, concentrated grape juice), dried apricots, rice flour, oat bran, cornmeal, brown rice syrup, barley malt, brown rice crisp, natural flavors, leavening.

Serving size: 1 bar	Sodium: 55 mg
Calories: 250	Carbohydrates: 50 grams
Fat: 2 grams	Fiber: 2 grams
Saturated fat: 0.5 gram	Sugars: 14 grams
Cholesterol: 0	Protein: 6 grams

BTU Stoker

Ingredients: Brown rice syrup, oat bran, natural fruit juice, milk protein (lactose-free calcium caseinate), crisped rice, dates, maltodextrin, natural cocoa powder, rice bran, almond butter, soy lecithin, natural chocolate, natural vanilla.

Serving size: 1 bar	Sodium: 70 mg
Calories: 250	Carbohydrates: 47 grams
Fat: 3 grams	Fiber: 4 grams
Saturated fat: 0.5 gram	Sugars: 16 grams
Cholesterol: 0	Protein: 10 grams

NUTS

Most conventional nuts are incredibly high in fat, but by roasting soybeans, corn, and other great foods, Sycamore Creek, based in Mason, Michigan, gives you a very healthy super-portable treat. You don't need utensils or cooking equipment, just a handful of these soybeans and all the nutrients are there. Inventor Leonard Stuttman believes that too many of our foods are overprocessed. He says, "I wanted to come up with a whole food that's tasty, minimally processed, palatable and digestible." The tradeoff is the fat content.

Roasted Soynuts — Salted

Ingredients: Soybeans, partially hydrogenated soybean oil, salt.

Serving size: 1 oz.	Sodium: 46 mg
Calories: 140	Carbohydrates: 8 grams
Fat: 7 grams	Fiber: 5 grams
Saturated fat: 1 gram	Sugars: 1 gram
Cholesterol: 0	Protein: 10 grams

Roasted Sweet Corn — Salted
Ingredients: Sweet corn, partially hydrogenated soybean oil, salt.

Serving size: 1 oz.	Sodium: 46 mg
Calories: 120	Carbohydrates: 20 grams
Fat: 5 grams	Fiber: 2 grams
Saturated fat: 1 gram	Sugars: 1 gram
Cholesterol: 0	Protein: 3 grams

Roasted Sunflower Seeds— Salted
Ingredients: Sunflower kernels, partially hydrogenated soybean oil, salt.

Serving size: 1 oz.	Sodium: 163 mg
Calories: 175	Carbohydrates: 4 grams
Fat: 16 grams	Fiber: 2 grams
Saturated fat: 2 grams	Sugars: 2 grams
Cholesterol: 0	Protein: 6 grams

Roasted Wheatnuts — Salted
Ingredients: Wheatberries, partially hydrogenated soybean oil, salt.

Serving size: 1 oz.	Sodium: 50 mg
Calories: 140	Carbohydrates: 16 grams
Fat: 6 grams	Fiber: 1 gram
Saturated fat: 1 gram	Sugars: 1 gram
Cholesterol: 0	Protein: 5 grams

COLD BREAKFAST CEREALS

This may seem impractical, but if you take along a box of super-high-fiber cereal, you can munch on it as you go. Ask for a carton of skim milk from the flight attendant or pick one up at a convenience store. Since this really loads you up on hunger-killing fibers, you can avoid a potholed road full of errors by taking a box on your next trip.

Arrowhead Mills Organic Puffed Kamut.
Ingredients: Puffed organic whole grain Kamut.

Serving size: 2 cups	Saturated fat: 0
Calories: 100	Cholesterol: 0
Fat: 0	Sodium: 0

Carbohydrate: 22 grams   Sugars: 0
Fiber: 4 grams   Protein: 4 grams

Arrowhead Mills Shredded Wheat
Ingredients: Organic whole wheat, natural vitamin E.

Serving size: 1 cup   Sodium: 0
Calories: 170   Carbohydrates: 41 grams
Fat: 0.5 gram   Fiber: 6 grams
Saturated fat: 0   Sugars: 0
Cholesterol: 0   Protein: 5 grams

Puffed Kashi
Ingredients: Whole oats, long-grain brown rice, whole rye, whole hard red winter wheat, whole triticale, whole buckwheat, whole barley, sesame seeds.

Serving size: 1 cup   Sodium: 0
Calories: 70   Carbohydrates: 16 grams
Fat: less than 1 gram   Fiber: 2 grams
Saturated fat: 0   Sugars: 0
Cholesterol: 0   Protein: 3 grams

★★ Arrowhead Mills Puffed Whole Millet
Ingredients: Puffed whole millet.

Serving size: 1 cup   Sodium: 0
Calories: 90   Carbohydrates: 19 grams
Fat: 0.5 gram   Fiber: 1 gram
Saturated fat: 0   Sugars: 0
Cholesterol: 0   Protein: 3 grams

Health Valley 98% Fat Free Granola (Date and Almond)
Ingredients: Oats, dates (coated with brown rice flour), molasses, brown rice flour, sprouted barley malt, pear-pineapple juice, concentrated grape juice, brown rice syrup, natural vanilla, rice bran, natural almond flavor, baking soda, sea salt.

Serving size: ⅔ cup   Saturated fat: 0
Calories: 180   Cholesterol: 0
Fat: 1 gram   Sodium: 90 mg

Carbohydrates: 43 grams   Sugars: 10 grams
Fiber: 6 grams   Protein: 5 grams

Cheerios

Ingredients: Whole grain oats, modified food starch, wheat starch, sugar, salt, oat fiber, trisodium phosphate, calcium carbonate, vitamin E.

Serving size: 1 cup   Sodium: 280 mg
Calories: 110   Carbohydrates: 23 grams
Fat: 2 grams   Fiber: 3 grams
Saturated fat: 0   Sugars: 1 gram
Cholesterol: 0   Protein: 3 grams

Fiber One

Ingredients: Wheat bran, corn bran, maltodextrin, corn starch, guar gum, caramel and annatto extract color added, cellulose gum, salt, baking soda, calcium carbonate, aspartame, and added vitamins and minerals.

Serving size: ½ cup   Sodium: 140 mg
Calories: 60   Carbohydrates: 24 grams
Fat: 1 gram   Fiber: 13 grams
Saturated fat: 0   Sugars: 0
Cholesterol: 0   Protein: 2 grams

CAMPING FOODS

These are the original dehydrated foods. This is a great way to eat really cheap and well on the road. If you're on a budget, as we are in the news business, you really can eat on ten dollars or less a day. Be sure to check out the sugar content, because these can be killers.

Martin Welch, Ph.D., discovered the need for dried, healthy, pure whole fruits and vegetables. He says, "We had a contract with the Department of Agriculture and needed to get ahold of some dried mango. We bought some from Thailand that was very sugared and tasted terrible — which was the kind of dried fruit available to Americans. Basically, we wasted our money. We said, 'We're scientists, we can do better than that.' We developed the mango that we now sell."

His four-year-old company, Kariba Farms, today offers consumers many varieties of dried fruits and vegetables including pineapples, strawberries, mangos, broccoli, carrots, red bell pepper, green bell pepper, and spinach, which can be eaten right out of the bag.

Kariba Farms Dried Mangos
Ingredients: Mangos, sodium metabisulphite for color.

Serving size: 40 grams	Sodium: 0
Calories: 120	Carbohydrates: 28 grams
Fat: 0	Fiber: 7 grams
Saturated fat: 0	Sugars: 19 grams
Cholesterol: 0	Protein: 1 gram

PICNIC: CREATE YOUR OWN SNACK FOOD

I soak beans overnight, then throw them into a cup and take them with me. This is as easy as it gets. Soybeans are sweet, chewy, and tasty. If you write or have to think, they're a great way to go. What I love about this is that you can keep a cup by your side and just pick away at it as much as you want. The more you eat, the healthier you are. It can't make you fat and will make you feel terrific. The other super-portable meal is a cup of low-fat, no-sugar yogurt added to a cup of uncooked oats. Add some apple, orange, or banana. It's great on an airplane, in a rental car, or at the office. The high-protein combo of oats and yogurt is super-energizing, and the high fiber is very filling. The big advantage of uncooked oats or oatmeal is that they have a much lower glucose load and much higher soluble-fiber load than cooked oatmeal.

COMPLETE MEALS

Amy's Kitchen of Petaluma, California, has created frozen meals without any chemical preservatives or additives. Their products say, "If you can't pronounce it, you won't find it on an Amy's label." Traditionally, frozen foods have tasted like repackaged airline dinners. But today, more frozen food items in natural food stores are being sold in grocery stores and supermarkets. And as time goes on they are getting tastier and tastier. This family-owned business's vision is frozen, great-tasting, wholesome, vegetarian food that can support a family's busy lifestyle. In fact, the idea was born along with founders Andrew and Rachel Berliner's daughter, Amy. Because there was little time to prepare wholesome, nutritious meals, their products were created for people like them looking for a hearty, home-cooked, tasty meal made with natural ingredients, but with the convenience of a frozen dinner. Here's a list of some of Amy's products as well as other meals I like:

Amy's Mexican Tamale Pie

Ingredients: Filtered water, organic pinto beans, organic tomatoes, organic corn, organic zucchini, organic cornmeal, onions, mochi rice flour, expeller-pressed safflower oil, cilantro, sea salt, and garlic.

Serving size: 8 oz.	Sodium: 480 mg
Calories: 220	Carbohydrates: 41 grams
Fat: 3 grams	Fiber: 11 grams
Saturated fat: 0	Sugars: 4 grams
Cholesterol: 0	Protein: 10 grams

Amy's Chicago Veggie Burger

Ingredients: Mushrooms, filtered water, organic tofu, onions, organic rolled oats, organic bulgur wheat, gluten flour, cheddar cheese (rennetless), organic brown rice, organic celery, organic carrots, organic walnuts, sea salt, organic potato flakes, organic garlic powder, expeller-pressed safflower oil.

Serving size: 2.5 oz.	Sodium: 390 mg
Calories: 160	Carbohydrates: 20 grams
Fat: 5 grams	Fiber: 4 grams
Saturated fat: 1.5 grams	Sugars: 2 grams
Cholesterol: 5 mg	Protein: 9 grams

Amy's Tofu-Vegetable Lasagna

Ingredients: Organic cooked lasagna pasta (organic semolina flour, organic whole wheat durum flour, water), organic tomatoes, onions, filtered water, mozzarella-style soy cheese (fresh soy milk made from organic soybeans and filtered water, soy oil, caseinate, fresh tofu, salt, soy lecithin, natural flavor, natural vegetable gums), organic zucchini, organic tofu, organic spinach, olive oil, organic carrots, spices, sea salt, and garlic.

Serving size: 9.5 oz.
Calories: 300
Fat: 10 grams
Saturated fat: 1 gram
Cholesterol: 0

Sodium: 630 mg
Carbohydrates: 41 grams
Fiber: 6 grams
Sugars: 6 grams
Protein: 18 grams

Amy's Black Bean and Vegetable Enchilada

Ingredients: Filtered water, tortilla (organic white corn cooked in water with a trace of lime), organic tomatoes, organic tofu, organic black beans, organic yellow corn, organic zucchini, mochi rice flour, expeller-pressed safflower oil, onions, organic bell peppers, spices, sea salt, tapioca flour, black olives, garlic, organic green chilies, and chives.

Serving size: 4.75 oz.
Calories: 130
Fat: 4 grams
Saturated fat: 0
Cholesterol: 0

Sodium: 390 mg
Carbohydrates: 20 grams
Fiber: 2 grams
Sugars: 1 gram
Protein: 4 grams

Fantastic Foods Original Grilled Nature's Burger

Ingredients: Vegetables (onions, mushrooms, carrots, zucchini, garlic), barley, oats, brown rice, red wheat, wheat gluten, lentils, soy sauce (water, wheat, soybeans, salt), brown rice syrup, carrageenan (seaweed extract), yeast extract, natural flavors, salt, spices.

Serving size: 1 patty
Calories: 120
Fat: 2 grams
Saturated fat: 0
Cholesterol: 0

Sodium: 290 mg
Carbohydrates: 23 grams
Fiber: 4 grams
Sugars: 3 grams
Protein: 7 grams

READ BETWEEN THE LINES: SOFT FAST FOODS

These foods appear to be hard fast foods, but on closer reading of the label they have fatal flaws. As educated consumers we need to be able to read between the lines. Here's a look at a few:

Bien Padre Foods Blue Organic Corn Tortilla Chips
Ingredients: Organically grown blue corn, high oleic safflower oil, sea salt.

Serving size: 1 oz.	Sodium: 70 mg
Calories: 150	Carbohydrates: 17 grams
Fat: 8 grams	Fiber: 4 grams
Saturated fat: 1 gram	Sugars: 0
Cholesterol: 0	Protein: 2

These chips look pretty good. They're packed with fiber and low in sugar. The problem is the fat. As soon as you expand this to a reasonable serving, 1½ ounces, you've got 12 grams of fat, 18 percent of your recommended daily input.

Benzel's Pretzel Bakery's Pennysticks Oat Bran All Natural Pretzel Nuggets
Ingredients: Unbleached wheat flour, oat bran, malt, soybean oil, salt, yeast.

Serving size: 1 oz.	Sodium: 170 mg
Calories: 110	Carbohydrates: 23 grams
Fat: 1 gram	Fiber: 1 gram
Saturated fat: 0	Sugars: 2 grams
Cholesterol: 0	Protein: 3 grams

This seems to be a great health food on the face of it and I was pleasantly surprised to see them on the airplane. The tipoff is low fiber; that means there really isn't much oat bran in it. When you look at the ingredient list, the lead ingredient is white flour, not oat bran.

part three *The Plan*

16

Feedforward Eating

At this point, you may think you need degrees in biochemistry, physiology, and genetic engineering just to order lunch and a Nobel Prize nomination to throw together a decent dinner for six. You don't. Feedforward eating pulls together all the principles of dropping your glucose load, cutting your hunger, and making your brain feel great into a simple daily eating plan.

Conventional Wisdom
Listen to your body.

LEAN
Seize control of your mind and body through the foods you eat.

ROAD MAP

This chapter lays out the reactionary, symptom-driven style of eating that makes many of us much fatter than we ever chose to be. As a solution, Feedforward Eating will teach you in what order and at what times of day to eat foods to maximally control your weight, your hunger, and your mood. The day is divided into zones, each of which is complete with its own meal plan to allow you to feel how you want when you want. For each zone there are multiple different meals that you can pick and choose to suit your own tastes and lifestyle.

REACTIVE EATING

Most of us have taught ourselves to eat by impulsive, knee-jerk reactions to the feelings of the moment. We react to symptoms, moods, and deficiencies that were created by past dietary errors. We're playing catch-up. Reactive eating makes us slaves to food. Our senses tell us what to eat. We sometimes don't stop eating until we're nauseatingly bloated, with buttons flying off our pants or skirts. We start eating because we have the jitters of a rock-bottom blood sugar, the dysphoria of a sagging serotonin level, or the hangover of a five-course dinner.

Reactive eating relies on primitive senses common to many lower forms of life. Who's smarter? You or some primordial instinct left over from when our ancestors were squids? Did you ever consider why most obesity studies are done on rats and mice? Researchers are looking for basic instincts, not any kind of advanced decision-making analysis. The classic cartoon version of reactive eating is of a rat running on a treadmill so it will be rewarded with food. Good rats learn quickly that they will be rewarded with food for correctly performing a task. But to condition these rats, scientists manufacture a situation where the rats are good and hungry so the food can be used as a reward. Many humans are trained like laboratory rats to reward themselves with food. They wait for fatigue, hunger, elation, depression, weakness, sleepiness, or anxiety to tell them when to eat, then reward themselves with high-fat, high-sugar foods. Eating becomes a game of never-ending catch-up where you respond to the moment rather than devising eating tactics for a far more successful day.

Allowing food to run your life this way is crazy! What if we waited until a car's fuel tank was empty before we reacted and filled the tank with more gas? Highways would be strewn with abandoned cars. In most other aspects of our lives we plan in advance, but when it comes to eating we let Mother Nature or Madison Avenue do the driving. You have a choice: Feed your brain and body what it needs before it asks or wait for it to strike back with a major retaliatory binge-driven food orgy.

FEEDFORWARD EATING

Had you been given a choice, would you want to have felt anxious, tired, fatigued, or lacking concentration? What if you could have chosen in advance exactly how you would want to feel? That's the principle of Feedforward Eating. Feedforward Eating relies on real intellect. Feedforward Eating is consuming the right foods in advance of a meeting, a workout, a nap, or concentrated intellectual effort so that you feel and perform exactly as you want. With Feedforward Eating, you plan your day according to how you want to feel at a given time or for a specific activity. You then eat foods that will make you feel the way you want when you want. Need to be more aggressive and alert for a big morning meeting? No problem. Want to recover faster from a tough workout? Easy! Need to relax and concentrate? Kid stuff. Want to feel more energetic during your evening workout? Done. Feedforward Eating takes the immense arsenal of foods that act as drugs and projects it powerfully forward in time, not unlike a great army projecting strength across a troubled region to prevent war. Athletes have practiced Feedforward Eating for years. Smart aerobic athletes will take a carbohydrate/protein beverage mixture just before they begin a long workout. The drink feeds the amino acid tyrosine into their brain for superior mental stamina and glucose into their muscles to push them harder, longer. Athletes couldn't "feel" in advance that they needed those specific fuels. Research showed them that the carbo/protein solution would work. When they looked at their stopwatches and odometers, they confirmed that they had indeed gone faster and farther.

Some of the nation's leading business executives, who have gotten an advance look at this book, are already practicing Feedforward Eating and adding many productive hours of work to their already busy days. You can project forward in time performance improvements for work or play that improve concentration, creativity, and stamina. Unfortunately, many of the foods that we eat have real performance benefits that we are simply unaware of and are misplaced in our daily schedule. For example, we might take milk, a protein energizer, at bedtime, falsely believing it will help us sleep. That's the price we pay for not understanding the principles of Feedforward Eating. By staking out in advance exactly how you would like to feel and perform, you can extract the maximum amount out of foods. In this way you can redirect your body's physiology toward that of weight loss, kill your hunger before you become hungry, and make your brain feel great so that depression, anxiety, restlessness, craving, or bingeing don't ruin your day and your diet.

The reason Feedforward Eating works so well is this: The brain's natural craving for foods is to meet specific needs to make hormones, neurotransmitters, replace spent fuel stores, or rebuild damaged muscle. By the time you crave nutrients to meet those needs, you've already suffered a serious deficiency. The body signals you with urgent warnings that force you to overcorrect, which means overeat.

HOW TO START

Feedforward Eating begins with individually crafted meals, which are spaced at strategic intervals. With Feedforward Eating, you eat before the sight and smell of food or the pangs of hunger manipulate you to make disastrous food errors. To fully understand that, in each zone below, there is a direct comparison of reactive meals contrasted to Feedforward meals, the culinary version of goofus and gallant. The reactive meal is an attempt to right yourself after food blunders have capsized your day, offering reward or relief for the proceeding period of intense hunger or craving you have suffered through. To avoid the disaster of a reactive meal, you need steely resolve — or you can preempt those hungers and cravings with a Feedforward meal. The latter requires only the most modest amount of willpower since you've chosen in advance of anticipated needs. If you make that choice at breakfast, you set up your day so that you are empowered to make the right choice because of the immediate reward that allows you to act and feel the way you want to.

The following section orders engineered meals in a sequence that fits your activity schedule like a glove. You'll feel alert, active, and ready to go in the morning; composed for an afternoon of intense concentration; and relaxed enough to wind down in the evening. The heart of a designer day is the ability to prepare the body physically to shed fat overnight when your body has its best opportunity. Each zone is programmed to account for the principles of the chapters: maintaining a steady insulin level, killing hunger, and making the brain feel great.

Like most other red-blooded Americans, I find that Thanksgiving and Christmas dinners somehow end up around my waist. The scale registers five to eight pounds more after the holidays than it did in mid-November. I used to start in mid-January on a winterlong recovery diet that never seemed to go anywhere. The most remarkable part of Feedforward Eating for me is that I can now take that extra weight off at will. Anytime. Anywhere. I just slot the right meals into the right zones and away goes the fat. No dieting, no starvation, no hunger. I just switch my physiology to weight loss and boom, the weight vanishes.

PRINCIPLES OF THE FEEDFORWARD DAY

The following plan incorporates all of the key weight-loss strategies you have encountered reading this book. Here are the highlights:

- An empty stomach is the most efficient drug delivery system since it sits ready to transmit the messages you'd like to send to your brain.
- Protein power: The tyrosine in protein solves the first problem you face every morning: making your brain wake up. You can do that in a cruel and jolting way by slamming it with caffeine, a cigarette, and a bagel-induced sudden rush of blood sugar, or you can let it gently surge to life. Both approaches achieve the same result, although the first is short-lived, the latter lasts all day. When protein feeds tyrosine to the brain, you get a kinder, gentler form of adrenaline boost that makes your brain become alert and mentally sharp, and increases your concentration. This will give you a very big edge up on your day. Since your body's natural craving for carbohydrate is in the morning, a high-protein breakfast is a great preemptive strategy. Here's how to use protein as a drug. First, you want an empty stomach so the protein can gain rapid entry into your bloodstream. Second, you want the protein in a quickly digested form. Protein supplements, milk, soy powder, and yogurt are key examples. Third, you want the protein to be isolated from other foods long enough to exert its effect. I'll have a protein shake or glass of milk first thing in the morning, then allow it to settle at least 15 minutes before eating anything else. If you overpower the protein with carbohydrate,

you'll dilute the effect. Also, if you've overeaten the night before, you'll still have the lingering effects of the meal and grogginess from the hormonal effects of overeating that will make the protein largely ineffective. High-protein sources such as whey protein, milk, soy protein, and nonfat, no-sugar yogurt are best. From midmorning through midafternoon keep your protein intake high. That means at least 2 ounces of protein for every five ounces of carbohydrate. Use protein at the beginning of all meals to kill your hunger.

• Carbo power: Eat good low-glucose carbos such as high-fiber breakfast cereals to gear up for the day ahead. Be certain to eat your breakfast carbos about 15 minutes after a good hit of protein. Otherwise, you'll find that pure carbos can make you sleepy. Try to avoid overloading on carbos for breakfast and lunch since they'll cut down on your productivity. Late afternoon is when most of us feel we need a carbo pick-me-up. Assume you'll need at least twenty minutes for healthy carbos to kick in, so plan for it. If you know that at four o'clock every afternoon you feel a little restless and agitated and can't concentrate, plan to eat your carbos at 3:30 P.M. That way you prevent yourself from hurting your brain. Remember that carbohydrate cravings later in the day are not the natural cravings directed by the brain, but cravings induced by fatigue, stress, and caffeine. More carbos and less protein is also important to help with sleep.

How Much Carbohydrate to Eat

It's not quantity that counts but the ratio of carbos to protein. By decreasing the protein in a given meal and increasing the amount of carbohydrate, you facilitate the entry of tryptophan into the brain. Five ounces of carbos to one ounce of protein is enough if eaten on an empty stomach. Eating smaller meals that are prepared for a specific effect on your mood and well-being far outdistances the usual helter-skelter mishmash of junk found in our stomachs. You'll find those smaller meals more satisfying and an ideal way to control your weight. Just because it's a smaller meal, doesn't mean it can't be satisfying for many hours. By small meal, I mean small in calories. In fact, it might be a very bulky meal with lots of hard foods and fibers. If you pile in the right ingredients, that food will sit in your stomach and upper intestine for four to six hours.

If you eat carbos on a full stomach, though, don't expect much effect because they are diluted by other foods. Although you could pour huge amounts of highly refined carbos onto a full stomach to overpower the other contents in your stomach, that's exactly how we become really fat. As an example, after a big fatty meal, you could eat an enormous hot fudge sundae with tons of goop and you would make more serotonin. However, you'd be better served by planning in advance when you want the calming effects of carbohydrates to kick in, and then eating a small amount on an empty stomach.

- Fiber power: Pack your lunch and afternoon snacks with fiber to kill your hunger during the key fat-craving period. Then if your willpower breaks down, you're still full of great foods to buffer you against excess consumption. Beans have the most fiber power, followed by high-fiber breakfast cereals. Both give you a major dose of fiber without much carbohydrate. The Canyon Ranch also recommends you eat protein and fiber every time you eat a significant amount. Says Kathleen Johnson, M.S., R.D., program director of the nutrition department, "This will slow down the absorption of sugar into the blood and avoid the peaks and valleys that destroy equilibrium. We really believe in the glucose load and that it is an important factor to be reckoned with."
- Beat your hormones: The hormones that drive you to eat peak at certain hours. By eating strategically, you can prevent those hormones from overpowering your ability to choose the right foods. Low-fat lunches are a key way of decreasing galanin, the hormone in your brain that causes a severe craving for fat.
- Kill your hunger: Although specific foods kill your hunger, the strategic alignment of foods and meals goes the furthest to curing your hunger.
- Give your brain a great day: Your brain wants a varied day. It wants time for accumulating information, interfacing with other people, reflection, creativity, sleep, and recovery.
- Bean power: Beans three times a day give you the ultimate fiber, filling, and energizing power.
- Keep glucose loads low: This kills hunger and keeps you thin.

FEEDFORWARD ZONES

The Feedforward day is divided into five zones. Success in one zone sets up success in the next. A fumble in one zone sets up failure in the next. You won't have the usual cravings, symptoms, or hungers that drive you to eat, but you will learn to expect and enjoy the effects of those foods on your mood, performance, and hunger. As that happens, you'll know you're succeeding. You'll feel exactly the way you planned to and, unless you're a professional hypochondriac, chances are you won't plan to feel grumpy, irritable, or fatigued. You can fumble in noncritical zones and recover easily. But if you fumble in a critical zone, you could set the fuse for a real food frenzy. Since the confluence of the modern workday and your hormonal cycles set up the worst potential for food craving, food abuse, overeating, and bingeing in the late afternoon, you must lay a super-solid foundation early in the day. Overeating in the late afternoon in turn damages the evening and night zones so you blow the chance to lose weight overnight or to awake fresh enough to make the right food choices the following morning. To be blunt, your evening preparations determine your overall success or failure.

WHAT TO EAT

In each zone, I have suggested the key foods you need to eat. Add bulk to those, and fruits, vegetables, and other foods to round out your meal. To make life easy for yourself, remember that each of us only has about ten favorite meals. By learning to shop for, cook, and enjoy ten new meals, you will have transformed yourself. It's no more complicated than that. All of the changes in this book will become automatic as you simply slot a new Feedforward meal in place of an old feedback meal.

Use monotony to your advantage by not complicating your food choices. Find which meals work in a certain time period, then don't be afraid to rely on the same great meals over and over. If you have too much diversity, your plan becomes too hard to stick with. If you want to try different foods, experiment at lunch when you have the most time to recover. Above all, plan what you are going to have in advance. That will dampen the temptation to eat badly and will give you steely resolve. You don't need elaborate recipe suggestions. That comes later, once you've proved to yourself that the raw food ingredients really work. Then you can dress up your meals with flavorings,

Feedforward Zones

Zone	Meals
Power	Breakfast and morning snack
Preemptive	Lunch
Craving	Afternoon snack
Relaxation	Dinner
Fat	Nighttime snack

spices, herbs, sauces, veggies, fruits, even fat, as long as it's olive or canola oil.

I. THE POWER ZONE

Time line: Waking to lunch

BREAKFAST

Breakfast sets up your day for success or failure. When you first get out of bed, your blood sugar level is at its lowest for the day, often averaging around 60, well below a normal blood sugar of over 100. The right breakfast gets your blood sugar out of the basement so you can think straight and makes the brain neurotransmitters that make you alert and ready to charge into the new day. Most dieters set themselves up for failure before they leave the house for work by eating a terrible breakfast or none at all, creating hunger, fatigue, and stress. A great breakfast charges up your metabolism to burn calories throughout the day.

Reactive Breakfast 1

Running on fumes: This has become the breakfast of choice for almost everyone trying to control weight. By fumes, I mean relying on whatever food is in your gut from the previous evening. Your blood sugar can take hours to force itself up to the point that you can think clearly. Without food, your metabolism turns over at the speed of a turtle, which turns all of the fat-sucking hormones into overdrive.

Reactive Breakfast 2

Carbo high: The pulse of modern life pushes you against the grain of all your natural body rhythms to get up and out the door in the morning at full steam, before your body's ready. That presses you to feel great quickly and to get your blood sugar up into the normal operating zone. Toast, bagels, pancakes, cornflakes, most of the traditional breakfast foods cause a major overshoot in blood sugar because they are fast-burning carbos. Since your body knows their effects are short-lived, you're pressed to overeat them. Sure you'll be pumped, but several hours later your blood sugar falls through the floor. If you're a coffee drinker, the barrage of adrenaline from your falling blood sugar combined with caffeine will have many jittery by mid-morning. You had a great fifteen minutes, a terrible late morning, and now you're being driven into lunch famished.

Reactive Breakfast 3

Down on the farm: A high-fat breakfast of eggs, bacon, and sausage will set up daylong craving for more fat by signaling the brain to make more of the fat-craving hormone galanin. That's a pity, because our body doesn't crave fat in the morning, so the high-fat breakfast is building a craving at the time of day when you wouldn't otherwise have one.

Feedforward Breakfast 1

Protein punch: Shot out of the barrel with the right foods makes for a terrific day every day, with the fortitude to make the right choices at each ensuing meal. First eat protein to get your brain feeling good. On an empty stomach, that's easy to do. A glass of skim milk, whey, or soy protein powder will work fastest.

As soon as you get out of bed, go to the refrigerator and pour yourself a glass of milk. Drink it before brushing your teeth, showering, or changing. As you shower and get dressed for work, the protein will perform its magic. There's enough lactose in the milk to get your blood sugar rising as well. When you're dressed and ready for breakfast, the protein will have dampened your appetite. Now plan to eat a super-hard, low-glucose carbo to ease yourself into the day and supply long-lasting energy. This is the base that will kill your appetite until lunch. A good hard morning carbo is a home-cooked, high-fiber oatmeal. Don't be afraid to add a little brown sugar. The oatmeal is so filling that the little bit of extra flavoring sugar won't do you any harm. To add bulk, have half a cantaloupe. This is the top-rated fruit for minerals, vitamins, and antioxidants. That's it. That's all you need for breakfast. Any more food is overkill. Now be patient. Your blood sugar will climb into the normal zone and sit there all morning long without faltering and without any overshoot. Get used to a calm, relaxed, vigilant state to replace the wired state of a reactive breakfast. Try as best you can to avoid early morning caffeine and let your foods wake you up and get you going. Fruit juice doesn't make much sense. The fructose won't raise your low fasting blood sugar to get your brain functioning for the morning ahead. You'll get more nutrients by having the real thing.

Feedforward Breakfast 2

Hard core: If you're too pressed for time to eat breakfast, make up a shake to run out the door with. I'll add Met Rx to some Fiber One cereal with a banana, ice, and water. In a hotel room, you can mix the Met Rx in the ice container, drink it, and run. ★★★★

Feedforward Breakfast 3

Beaten not stirred: Here's a way to resuscitate the big breakfast for days when you have time to sit down to relax and have a nice breakfast. An omelette prepared with Egg Beaters or egg whites only, low-fat cheese, onions, tomatoes, and mushrooms, but without the butter, cream, or whole milk provides a nice slow-burning meal that will kill your hunger for much of the morning and give you enough calories to get your metabolism going. This is a reasonable way to go. ★★★

Feedforward Breakfast 4

Fiber One: OK, so I've stolen the name from a food company, General Mills to be specific. This is the easiest possible way to get a huge hit of fiber early in the day to act as a satiator. One brimming bowl gives you an unbelievable amount of fiber, 13 grams. In fact, three bowls gives you the full 35 grams that the American Cancer Society recommends. To load up on tyrosine, I like to have a glass of skim milk first, then have another glass in the Fiber One. A piece of fruit, and that's all you need. The chapter "Hard Fibers" lists the cereals that are highest in protein. Choose ones with the highest soluble fiber such as Kellogg's Heartwise, General Mills Benefit, Kolln Oat Bran Crunch, or Quaker Oat Bran Cereal. ★★★★★

Feedforward Breakfast 5

Mediterranean morning: Nancy Jenkins, nationally known food writer and author of *The Mediterranean Diet Cookbook,* suggested this terrific breakfast from the world's healthiest culture. Start with nonfat yogurt, then eat a dense, grainy, coarse bread, toasted. The bread should be a firm multigrain bread.

Feedforward Breakfast 6

Mexican motivator: Arline D. Salbe, Ph.D., R.D., the research nutritionist for the National Institutes of Health, National Institute of Diabetes and Digestive and Kidney Diseases, Clinical Diabetes and Nutrition Section in Phoenix, Arizona, suggests starting with plain fat-free yogurt topped with fresh strawberries. Then have a whole wheat burrito stuffed with three cooked egg whites and chopped green chilies, wrapped in a whole wheat fat-free tortilla.

Feedforward Breakfast 7

Chang Mai Hai: The Thais make wonderful use of limited fats and sugars as ways of inducing you to eat great foods. It is the premier culture for doing so and thereby cutting glucose load. I ordered a Thai omelette for breakfast in Chang Mai last winter. Inside was a delightful chicken, rice, and pea meal with a slightly sweet sauce. The *"xteriro,"* as they call the omelette, was made of egg but was paper thin. This gave you the great mouth feel of fat and the taste of a crave-killing sweet. You could eat your fill, knowing that you had great hunger-killing, super-filling foods with just that trace of fat and sweetness. As you eat such an omelette, you realize what overkill an American omelette is, so densely packed with fats. At the end of your Thai meal, your stomach is light, not heavy.

Feedforward Breakfast 8
Mountain high: Here's an amazingly portable, super-energizing breakfast. Mix one cup of low-fat, no-sugar yogurt with uncooked oats. Add some grated apples, orange slices, and banana. I love to brown-bag this super-portable breakfast onto early morning flights.

MIDMORNING SNACK
Reactive Midmorning Snack 1
Dull as donuts: This meal is a reaction to low blood sugar, either because you never ate at all or because your blood sugar has crashed. The knee-jerk reaction to this condition is a fast-burning sugar. At midmorning in Manhattan I see dozens of people lined up for donuts, sticky buns, and bagels. The damage is doubled when a sugar-starved and -addled brain reaches out for as many calories as it can get. Since your stomach feels really empty, you may feel you have the extra latitude to eat lots. Your stomach will empty quickly, so you become a bottomless hole into which you can dump pounds of bakery goods. The fat cranks up your craving for more and more. That's why donuts and sugar-covered fatty bakery items lead the list of bad midmorning snacks. When your blood sugar crashes again, you'll feel like a dope.

Feedforward Midmorning Snack 1
Mexican standoff: Keep the ratio of protein to carbohydrate high. Look for foods high in soluble fibers. I eat a black bean and corn salad.

Feedforward Midmorning Snack 2
Battle Creek: A single bowl of high-fiber cereal will decrease your risk of heart disease by 20 percent and give you 10 grams of fiber. I eat this midmorning with a glass of skim milk. It's a terrific low-calorie filler.

Feedforward Midmorning Snack 3
Hard core: A cup of soybeans are an ideal way to punch up your alertness and fill you to the brim.

2. THE LOADING ZONE
Time line: Lunch through late afternoon

LUNCH

Lunch makes a pivotal difference in the productivity of your afternoon. It can keep you on a roll or deaden your afternoon by launching you into an early and lengthy siesta-like stupor. Kathleen Johnson, M.S., R.D., of the Canyon Ranch, says, "People don't feel real good when the meal is made up mostly of carbohydrate. My experience is that if you have more protein at lunch, you will feel better in the afternoon. Basically, what we've gleaned from the literature and our experience is that a meal that is a bit higher in protein seems to result in feelings of alertness. A meal of fish and a lot of vegetables seems a lot less likely to cause you to doze off in the afternoon than a lot of pasta will.

Reactive Lunch 1
1950s replay: A big heavy meat lunch of steak or veal makes your blood milky and cloudy with high levels of fats. The sheer number of calories keeps your insulin high. You won't be hungry, but the lunch was overkill. The insulin and fat combination will give you the girth a sumo wrestler would be proud of.

Reactive Lunch 2
Pasta heaven: The 1950s' three-martini lunch was clearly a killer, but the much-vaunted pasta lunch has become its replacement. The pasta's medium-glucose carbs will make you sleepy and dull during the afternoon. You'll be famished by late afternoon when your blood sugar falls.

Reactive Lunch 3
Sparrow's pickings: You feel oh so pious that you've slid through the day without breakfast and escaped from lunch with some leafy greens and a carrot. Don't be fooled. A tidal wave of hormone-driven craving is descending on you as your fat cells get ready to suck up anything that comes their way.

Reactive Lunch 4
Airline anything: This is fiber-free eating at its best, whether it's the New York–Washington shuttle with bagel and cream cheese, a linguine lunch, or chicken and mashed potatoes, you will be hard served to get *any* fiber on an airplane. That will leave you plenty hungry at the conclusion of dinner. That's why I always fall for the ice cream sundae on the transcontinental flights . . . I'm starved. Bring along anything from the "Hard Fast Foods" chapter and you'll protectively fill yourself up for the trip.

Feedforward Lunch 1
Shark attack: This is the time to fill 'er up, not with calories but with bulk. This is your best chance to avoid a big dinner by really laying in foods that will just sit in your stomach. Start with protein to keep yourself alert for the afternoon. If you can't drink milk, then consider a nice piece of fish or chicken. Order and eat your meat course before you touch another piece of food. Remember that protein is the great satiator and you want to give it a chance to satiate you and make your brain feel good. I'll have shark with a sweet potato and a papaya. Forget the water and pass on the bread. Then go for the carbos, but make certain they are slow burning so you stop after several hundred calories.

Feedforward Lunch 2
Veggie delight: In the nutritional minefield that our cafeteria has become, the one safe play is a veggie burger, heavy on the soybeans, with a hard seven-grain bread.

Feedforward Lunch 3
Bean blast: If there's no time for a hot meal, try black mung beans and bulgur, barley, or oats. You'll be hard pressed to believe you can remain so alert but remain so relaxed. Here's one meal that several glasses of water can expand to fill your stomach.

A properly balanced lunch still is high in protein with a modest amount of carbohydrates: too few carbos may leave you on edge, too many feels like the sandman. If you come into lunch from a great breakfast and midmorning snack, you won't feel like a big lunch. If you're worried about getting hungry during the afternoon, remember you've still got lots of snacking to do. By killing your hunger with a high-fiber bean blast, you cut the naturally high craving for fat that peaks soon after lunch.

Feedforward Lunch 4

Shoes of the fisherman: Arline Salbe, Ph.D, R.D., recommends fish tacos made with freshly grilled tuna chunks, shredded romaine lettuce, chopped fresh tomato, and shredded cabbage, all topped with a spicy low-fat dressing (salsa, no-fat yogurt, low- or no-fat mayo, pickle relish), served with fresh fruit.

Feedforward Lunch 5

Fiesta: Dr. Salbe also recommends chicken fajitas: white meat chicken marinated and grilled along with onions, red and green sweet peppers, and tomato chunks, wrapped in a whole wheat fat-free tortilla, and served with steamed brown rice, cooked black beans, and pico de galo (fresh tomato salsa) sauce.

3. THE CRAVING ZONE

Time line: Midafternoon

SNACK AND DINNER

Midafternoon is when your natural cravings for food hit their zenith. You're fighting a major urge to eat fat brought on by the highest levels of galanin. Any fat you eat will store quickly and fire up your appetite for even more fat. This is also afternoon delight time for carbohydrate cravers. Late afternoon is when we lose our concentration and get fidgety, even slightly dysphoric. Fast-burning carbos are the quick fix, but a fix we need to hammer ourselves with again and again to remain happy.

Reactive Snack 1

Candy counter: I can't tell you the number of times I've blown it in the craving zone. It's late afternoon, I have a news story we're "crashing" to get on the evening news. Candy bars, muffins, bagels, pies, cakes, or other high-carbo fat-laden food will satisfy the cravings but light the fuse that ruins your day. High-glucose carbos can send you on a food frenzy that won't end until bedtime. Since they go through your system so quickly, you'll feel light and hungry with no signal to stop. It's the ideal appetizer to pile through an enormous dinner or to get ready for that all-you-can-eat contest.

Feedforward Snack 1

Butch Cassidy's last stand: Think of four o'clock as time to build the dike. Beat your cravings by stuffing yourself with low-density, great-tasting foods that are part of a balanced meal of slow-burning carbos and protein. My favorite is a whole wheat quesadilla with black beans, brown rice, and a small amount of low-fat cheese. This will kill my appetite for dinner and fill me up through bedtime, which sets me up perfectly for the next morning. No matter how badly you messed up earlier in the day, this is your last great shot at recovery. You may think that a minimeal is overkill, but 200 to 400 calories well invested here can prevent a thousand into the evening. You'd be surprised that a good minimeal has fewer calories than a fatty muffin.

4. THE RELAXATION ZONE

Time line: Early evening

DINNER

The basic premise of dinner is false. You do not need to reload after a hard day at the office or with the kids unless you do heavy manual labor, like that advocated for inmates of southern prisons. Now that the bulk of your day is behind you and you're cutting down on activities, you should be cutting down on your fueling as well. The concept is simple: Fuel in advance of activities, not after they are completed. And if there is one activity you certainly never want to fuel for, it's sleep. If you do, you're using foods to send your brain confusing messages: Wake me up, keep me up, and make me fat. Your entire ability to control your weight is predicated on what you do after sundown. That's not to say that previous zones weren't important. The wrong foods earlier in the day strip away any control you should have over your evening. But if you can eat a dinner that kills your hunger efficiently and leaves your insulin level steady, you'll burn calories as you sleep and wake up lighter the next morning. Dumping extra calories into your body after dark sets up a cycle of weight gain.

Reactive Dinner 1

Broadway: If dining is the theater of the '90s, then large festive celebrations like wedding receptions, retirement dinners, fund raisers, and benefits are opening night on Broadway. I attended one such event last year determined to make all the right food choices. And I did, for most of the first hour. But by the time the twenty-seventh toast was proposed, the only decent way to entertain myself was with the wealth of food that was dumped on my plate, because the extemporaneous speeches just didn't cut it. Picture it. First the father toasts, followed by the son, the son's friend, the baby-sitter, roommates, classmates, lovers, uncles, cousins, grandparents, waiters, passersby. The food goes down faster and faster, eased by wine, sparkling water, champagne, table water until . . . boom! . . . you're cooked! When your head hits the sack, you can feel your intestine churning, kneading, sucking, and sloshing the remnants of your nightmare meal. Now, your body has a natural safeguard against extra calories; it increases oxidation. That means it begins burning more calories by turning up your metabolism, but hardly enough to prevent that extra fat from lining your midsection. As your gut churns and your metabolism roars, you will toss and turn enough to be the envy of even the most ambitious sleep-medication infomercial producer. You'll awaken groggy and either too full or too nauseated to eat breakfast. And it doesn't take your daughter's wedding to make it happen. You name it, from steak and mashers, burgers and fries, to fettucine Alfredo and pizza — if it's a big dinner, it's a killer.

Reactive Dinner 2

Hoover: Most Americans are smart enough to know that a big dinner makes them fat, so they graze through the evening. A better expression would be to vacuum or "hoover." If it's in the way, we mow right through it and suck it up: chips, frozen yogurt, leftover pizza, corn chips, cookies. After a fast-burning carbo snack in late afternoon, we're famished by the foods that never say no. Hunger is at red alert. When you exit the cheating zone with pent-up hunger, you are making yourself more vulnerable than at any other time of the day. On my son's eighth birthday, I made the cardinal error of eating a box of Milk Duds before coming home. On my arrival, our next-door neighbor offered me a piece of pumpkin pie. Gone. Then I discover my son's leftover birthday cake. Demolished. Three pieces of pizza left over from the baby-sitter. Hoovered. Yet I never felt full.

Feedforward Dinner 1

Land fill: A high-bulk dinner punctuated with high-soluble-fiber foods is your best protection. I like a whole wheat burrito with chicken, brown rice, and black beans. This fills your stomach to the stretching point with a modest number of calories.

Feedforward Dinner 2

Food of the fisherman: When you're forced to dine out, start with a piece of broiled fish. Insist on the fish before having your water poured. Send the bread basket back. Let the fish kill your hunger. Then order the rest of your dinner. With your appetite vanished, you'll have a commanding control over your waiter. Now go for the sweet potato, whole rice, beans, and veggies. *Never* go to dinner without your afternoon meal, which you should use to kill your hunger through dinner.

Feedforward Dinner 3: Eating Out

Intestinal condoms: One huge error we make when eating out is to go out hungry figuring we're going to try to be good but will probably eat a lot anyhow. Wrong! You should always use a little prophylaxis. By eating high-fiber hard foods, you are laying down a special coating of a gumlike gel along the walls of your intestine. This slows the absorption of nutrients. Hard foods also increase satiety, so you have the chance to avoid a huge meal. I'll have a big brown rice and bean plate before I head out in the evening. Now even if you don't eat less food, you'll find that your control is enormously enhanced so that the foods you eat are safe, health-making foods. You'll have the presence of mind, the willpower, and self-esteem to really choose.

Balance: By increasing the amount of protein in your dinner, you increase your vigilance and alertness. If you have a big evening where you have to give a speech or stay up late, you'll need to continue with this higher amount of protein. The fish dinner will do that nicely. But if you need to kick back or relax, then you'll want to do more carbos. That's where I like beans and grains.

Feedforward Dinner 4

Canyonlands: Evening is the best time to make a concentrated effort to eat your veggies. At the Canyon Ranch, nutritionists have had great success making the evening meal a vegetarian meal. The high-carbo content gives you a good shot of serotonin to calm down, while the low glucose load assures a good night's sleep by keeping your insulin from spiking.

Duke's mix is a super-efficient way of getting all your veggies in one big gulp. It's the favorite combination of vegetables of Dr. James Duke, the pioneer of foods as medicine. Throw the following vegetables in a Vita-Mixer for 90 seconds at high speed to make two cups.

- 2–4 tomatoes
- 1 or 2 sweet red or green peppers
- Hot pepper — any type jalapeño is fine — for the antioxidant capsaicin
- Whole onion (with skin — it's the richest source of the antioxidant quercetin)
- ½ cup kale and/or turnip greens or collards
- 1–4 carrots (fresh)
- 1 cup purslane, a common weed found at most farmer's markets
- 1 or 2 spears of broccoli

Feedforward Dinner 5

The all-American: Here's another dinner from the Canyon Ranch for those evenings out where you have to eat a full meal. Start with a modest serving of salmon. Then go for a full cup of vegetables and a modest serving of brown rice or sweet potato.

Feedforward Dinner 6
Mediterranean: Nancy Harmon Jenkins, author of *The Mediterranean Cookbook,* recommends a frittata omelette made with a mixture of whole eggs and egg whites, fresh mint, and onions; small coarse bread rolls, called *friselle,* piled with chopped tomatoes, arugula, and an oil and vinegar dressing, accompanied by a glass of red wine. For dessert: a handful of green almonds and a few cherries with honey.

Feedforward Dinner: Dessert
Sweet craving: Once you're completely full, you may still have a real craving for sweets. You may choose to persevere and allow that craving to disappear over several weeks' time. However, if it's just killing you, try this. Suck on just two pieces of milk chocolate, which may do far more to satisfy your craving than three pieces of cake with frosting. Here's why. Cake, ice cream, cookies, and other desserts will take a long time to work their way through your digestive system to give you the druglike hit your sweet tooth is craving. If you've eaten a meal with really slow-burning carbos, then you'll have to eat a tremendous amount of cake to budge your blood sugar up to the point you are satisfied. However, recall that when you eat a piece of chocolate, there is a communications pathway directly from your mouth to your brain that will give you the rush of endorphins you're looking for immediately, without waiting for your body to digest it. A full stomach should prevent you from overdosing. Concentrate on feeling the chocolate hit, then sit back and enjoy it. Your craving should subside. Be careful not to take more than a panel or two from a Hershey Bar, or the caffeine in the chocolate may keep you awake. Allow the chocolate to melt in your mouth, under your tongue, rather than eating it.

5. THE FAT ZONE
Time line: Night

LOSE WEIGHT OVERNIGHT!
Three-quarters of the world's population goes to bed hungry, and so should you. I don't mean the gut-searing hunger that keeps you awake; however, your stomach should feel nearly empty as you fall

asleep. This will set you up perfectly for burning fat overnight. The first several nights you try this, you'll notice your weight is about a pound lighter on the scale the following morning. Here's why. As your body looks for fuel to burn overnight, it can take it directly from your undigested dinner or it can pull it from fat stores. With an empty stomach and a low insulin level, your body will select the fuel from your fat stores. With a big meal sitting in your stomach and a high insulin level, it will do exactly the opposite and store fuel as fat. If you remain full overnight, you'll kill your urge to eat breakfast, the meal that puts you back into the fat-burning mode. Since this is the longest stretch of time that we don't eat, it's the most important to prepare for, but we tend to pay this period the least amount of attention, thinking that it just won't matter. By tapering the amount you eat at dinner and afterwards, you assure yourself of an empty stomach when you sleep. Still the foods you do eat are terribly important for recovery and repair of tissue, quality sleep, restocking the neurotransmitters, and waking up in good cheer.

I call this the fat zone because it's when the floodgates into fat cells burst open. Here's why. After dark, most Americans consume the majority of their calories. They've tried to be good all day long. But the idea of being good often means no breakfast, a light lunch, and a killer afternoon snack. This puts our fat cells into starvation mode, hoovering anything that hits the palate. With fat and carbohydrate cravings at a maximum, this constellation of events pours over a thousand of exactly the wrong calories into a system loaded with increasing levels of insulin. Overnight, the flood of fat continues to pour fat into fat cells. We think we were being good because we remember the starvation, the emptiness, the hunger, but the next morning the scales don't lie: we're fatter. But getting fat overnight isn't the only downside. While a great night's sleep restores mood-enhancing neurotransmitters for a fresh start the following day, by spiking your insulin level with fast-burning carbos or a big meal before bedtime, your neurotransmitter stores don't refill, so you wake up groggy and starved for sleep. That's the revolutionary theory of Dr. Barry Sears, author of *The Zone*.

The last meal before you sleep sets up the hormonal and neurochemical foundation for the following day. "Remember," says Dr. Sears, "you're going through at least an eight-hour cycle. One thing you're looking to prevent is nocturnal low blood sugar. You don't want a big meal. You want a small snack with enough calories to generate hormonal responses that will eliminate nocturnal low blood sugar and more importantly, set the hormonal foundation for the maximum release of growth hormone that occurs during deep sleep."

Reactive 1

TV dining: Snack food is a great way to pile on major fat and fast-burning carbos. A bag of chips, some frozen yogurt, a cupcake. They don't seem like much, but blowing through 700 calories in the space of two prime-time shows is a snap.

Reactive 2

Have your cake: After a big dinner, some alcohol, and lots of water you've still got room for more . . . more candy, crackers, cookies, an extra piece of cake, leftovers from the fridge. You've eaten over half of your daily calories in the last several hours. You feel sleepy. After you hit the sack, your body is working overtime. With a sky-high insulin level, your body is packing that five-course dinner into one fat cell after another. Several hours later, you're wrestling in bed. Your heart goes thump, thump, thump. In the early morning hours you have a low blood sugar, bringing you out of any quality sleep you may have had and into a cold sweat.

Feedforward 1

The zone: In your weight-loss phase, if you've skipped dinner, try a small snack to control your hunger. The snack should contain no more than 100 calories that have the right balance of protein and carbohydrate. I avoid really hard foods so my digestive system isn't on overdrive when I'm trying to sleep. Dr. Barry Sears recommends two ounces of low-fat cottage cheese and half a piece of fruit. This gives you the hunger-killing, insulin-lowering effects of protein. I find some cheeses keep you awake. If that's true for you, try the following.

Feedforward 2

Late breakfast: Robert Pritikin told me: "Go to bed hungry. For a good night's sleep, eat a small high-carbo meal before bedtime." Breakfast cereals usually fit the bill. Both MIT's Dr. Judith Wurtman and Harvard's Dr. George Blackburn advocate the use of breakfast cereal in the evening. Dr. Blackburn says of his patients he puts on a diet, "They put breakfast cereal into that evening slot. They love it. And they get a big bowl and mix raisin bran and cornflakes. They have fun with it, they've got to."

I've tried this and found it very satisfying. It's light on the stomach, so you aren't kept awake at night, plus it's easy on your insulin so you don't wake up groggy. Try different combinations. Mix and match. I like Wheat Chex. Just look for cereals with more than 5 grams of fiber and less than 5 grams of sugar. Both fiber and sugar are clearly labeled on the FDA nutritional label required on the side of every cereal box. If you want to sweeten the cereal, sprinkle it with a higher GI index cereal such as Honey Nut Cheerios. You'll get used to a really light feeling in your stomach at night. On those occasions when you have a big dinner, you'll feel unnaturally full. You want the snack to be easy on the stomach and easy to digest, which is why breakfast cereals fit the bill. You can eat the cereal dry or add a small amount of milk, cottage cheese, or yogurt. That cuts the glucose load to keep your insulin low. At the Pritikin Center, eliminating caffeine and alcohol entirely also contributes to a much better night's sleep.

By following the guidelines of Feedforward Eating, you hasten the speedy exit of fats from their cozy home in fat cells out into your bloodstream so the body can consume them as fuel during the night. You may notice that it's harder than usual to wake up the next morning, because you've fallen into a much deeper sleep than your body is used to. That's good news because you'll look forward to breakfast as an energizer and wake 'er upper that will bring new vitality to your day. By preparing the previous evening with low-calorie, light meals and snacks, you are hungry enough in the morning so that you can eat exactly what you should. You'll be a far tougher food-decision maker earlier in the day and can keep that toughness with you. You'll notice that a Feedforward day may not look strikingly different from a reactive day, nor may it be much lower in calories in its planning stages (before the reactive eater overeats). Look at the following meal. Many savvy dieters would assume that this is an excellent example of an effective menu.

Reactive Day
Breakfast: one bagel
Lunch: turkey sandwich on sourdough bread
Snack: fat-free pretzels, Twizzlers, and SnackWell cookies
Dinner: pasta with red sauce and Italian bread

That's not a lot of food. Many dieters eat few calories, but those calories inflict maximum damage. Here's how the Canyon Ranch modifies that day, incorporating the feedforward principles.

Feedforward Day
Breakfast: bran flakes with skim milk and fruit
Lunch: keep the turkey sandwich at lunchtime but add dense
    whole grain bread
Snack: Nile Spice or Fantastic Foods instant bean soup with an apple
Dinner: a modest serving of salmon, a good full cup of vegetables,
    and a modest serving of brown rice or sweet potato

6. THE WORKOUT ZONE

The workout zone can be inserted into any part of your day. Since it will reduce your requirement for insulin, speed your metabolism, and jack up your brain's endorphins, it gives a natural boost to any weight-loss activities and serves as a great meal substitute.

Here's the logic behind most workouts: "Gee, I'm burning calories to lose weight, so I would be pretty silly to eat." However, the chances are good that we've taken a good load of fast-burning carbos on board in the hours before exercise, but have neglected to eat specifically to improve our workout. Most wrecked workouts result from a rapidly falling blood sugar caused by these fast-burning sugars in the diet. When you hop on the treadmill and feel your legs go wobbly, your brain grow blank, and your body bead with cold perspiration, you know you've "tanked" or "bonked," e.g., dropped your blood sugar level in the toilet. It's strong negative reinforcement for exercise and is a major reason that people get turned off from exercise. But don't be bummed. Even Olympic athletes ruin their training and competition by running high blood sugar and insulin levels before the gun goes off. In fact, the athletes' diets are extraordinarily hard on their systems. Olympians can seriously damage their coronary arteries despite the fact they are in vigorous training. Many of these athletes would perform a lot better and live far longer if they practiced Feedforward Eating. If you find that your workouts are lagging, especially during the weight-loss phase of a diet plan, consider the following:

Time line

Morning: The best all-round day begins with a workout. As the first activity of the day, you'll get a natural and long-lived energy explosion that no amount of food or caffeine can match. Your own hormones won't bring your body into peak performance until afternoon. This way you gain two performance peaks to your day. The only downside of a morning workout is that you can't push your body quite as hard as you can in the afternoon.

Afternoon: This is a great way to reward your brain with endorphins without having to resort to chocolates and fats. Inserted into the late afternoon doldrums, you can use the workout instead of a meal to cruise through the craving zone. A hard workout will kill your appetite for dinner.

Night: Mild aerobic exercise is a great way to prepare your body for sleep. Heavier aerobic and anaerobic exercise can make it very hard to go to sleep, so an easy workout is best. If you burn the midnight oil, an early evening workout will keep your energy going until the oil runs dry.

Reactive 1

The American dream: Over the long haul, any high-sugar, high-fat diet diverts fuel away from your muscle so that it's running on empty. The cell membranes transport sugars poorly into muscle with a high saturated-fat diet. High insulin levels divert the fuel away from muscle and into fat stores. A high-fat, high-sugar diet is death to workouts and, one day, the athlete as well.

Reactive 2

Carbo misloading: "Gosh, I've got a workout this afternoon. I'd better carbohydrate-load." In the hour or two before exercise you deliberately fill up on bagels, breads, cereals, figuring that you'll be fully carbo-loaded. The only thing that will be loaded is your stomach, which will be uncomfortably full of dreck. That won't save you when your blood sugar falls.

Reactive 3

Gator chug-a-lug: Sports drinks are a fast way to get your blood sugar up. But if you drink them more than fifteen minutes before a workout, you're asking for a short and ugly workout since your blood sugar is likely to crash.

Reactive 4

The full Clinton: This is the ability to erase completely any weight-loss benefits of a workout by reloading with burgers and fries at fast-food restaurants after the end of exercise.

Feedforward 1

Rocket fuel: The whole Feedforward program will lower your insulin levels and your body fat so that exercise becomes easier and easier and thus you are truly fired up for exercise. But to truly light the fuse on a great workout, take a motivator. Drink a protein-laced carbohydrate beverage three or four minutes before you begin an aerobic workout. Any longer and you risk dumping your blood sugar. The mixture I like is about 75 grams of carbos with 15 grams of whey protein. I reserve this maneuver for the two days a week I want a really hard workout of at least sixty minutes in length.

Feedforward 2

Power oats: Bill Evans, Ph.D., of the Noll Physiologic Research Center at Penn State University, has demonstrated that eating oats forty-five minutes before a workout also delivers a stronger, faster, longer workout. This is a better maneuver for weight control because it's designed to keep your insulin steady. These should be whole oats or a really high-quality oatmeal. If you're serious about weight loss, favor "power oats" over "rocket fuel."

Feedforward 3

Legal speed: While excess caffeine is a blunder in other parts of the day, it has a strong biochemical effect benefiting exercise. Caffeine releases free fat acids to preferentially burn fat. Over the course of an hour, you'll burn off much of the caffeine buzz to give you a very low aftereffect profile. Dr. George Blackburn says, "Caffeine and sports drinks will make your workout the most fun you can imagine. I believe in it absolutely." There's an extra bonus: Intense exercise causes the brain to create special nerve growth factors that account for continuing clarity and mental dexterity later in life.

Hard Cuisine

You're staring at a plate of hard foods: soybeans, broccoli, and cabbage. Sure, they'll make you hard as a rock, but are you tough enough to eat them? Not many of us are, yet there are hundreds of cultures around the world in which hard foods are eaten successfully by transforming them into spectacular cuisines. That transformation has developed into a fine art over thousands of years of experimentation with herbs, spices, and food ingredients. Foods embody a culture's spiritual values and societal aspirations. The people believe in these foods. In no place do you see more vividly the concept of you are what you eat than when you travel to the developing world. From the high Himalayas and the Sierra Madre to the lakes of northern Kenya and the shores of Okinawa, you see lean, taut, elegant people who have become hard through the meals that they treasure. What a striking contrast to the Oktoberfest beer tents in Munich and the theme parks of Orlando, Florida, where you see visitors with fat packed so tightly it appears to pop out of the skin, giving rise to the European term "balloon people." The difference is not willpower or even activity, it is the meals they eat. Eight major studies worldwide of eating habits and weight in different cultures show that millions who ate more food actually weighed less. Remember that the deadly American diet comes from the dullest, least imaginative culinary countries in the world: Germany and England! No one brags about English food, not even the Brits. German food fell to such depths that Germany's president, Helmut Kohl, had to write a book to defend it. That's why I find it so terribly hard to understand what's so difficult about giving up the widely caricatured meat-and-potatoes American diet. It's like being asked to give up a brown rusted-out Dodge De Soto for an Aston-Martin. What's to give up? What's the attachment? What's the sacrifice? The export of the low-fiber, high-sugar, high-fat Western diet has been followed by an epidemic of heart disease, diabetes, and cancer that has outdistanced any great plague since the Middle Ages. Give it up!

Conventional Wisdom
Eat American, just limit the portions.

LEAN
Go native.

MULTICULTURAL EATING

Think it's crazy to take up cross-cultural eating? We do it every day by ordering Chinese takeout, pizza, sushi, and burritos. The problem is that we have Americanized those dishes to the point that they are reduced to refined flours dripping with fat . . . many far worse for your heart or waistline than a Mac and fries. Over several years, the Center for Science in the Public Interest has studied the American versions of the most popular foreign cuisines. Instead of finding great taste delights engineered from fine herbs, they too found foods packed with tons more fat than the worst fast foods. That was across the board from Mexican to Chinese to Italian foods.

Skeptics will tell you that these cultures are genetically thin and would do just as well on any diet. Boy, are they wrong. Look at the fat cats in the big cities of countries that have traditionally had the best diets and you will see an explosion in diabetes, obesity, and coronary artery disease as they adopt our Western diet in countries from Japan and China to Kenya and Saudi Arabia. The reward for abandoning the diet that Western culture has so firmly embraced is a spectacular adventure. As you travel from one land to another you will find a rich tradition of foods that span the history of man.

ROAD MAP

Feedforward Eating allows you a vast range of different meals to control your weight. However, once you have brought your weight to where you want it, you should consider that only by selecting and sticking with a single cuisine is there any real guarantee of maximal health and a long life. Here's why you should consider an entire meal package from a real culture. The research just hasn't been done on a helter-skelter à la carte menu of foods over a lifetime to be able to say that one particular food prevents cancer or heart disease or makes you live longer. But that can be said for the entire diet of an individual country.

As you'll read for each of the following cultures, there are well-documented life expectancies and rates of heart disease and cancer to judge the diet's benefits. Nutritionists are loath to talk about good foods and bad foods. For instance, they won't call red meat bad because there are very lean grades and even the world's healthiest diets use red meat as a garnish. They believe that there are as yet unknown factors in the different foods that interact with each other to make a diet super-healthy. That is what has been so terribly wrong about the media approach to food — identifying public food enemy number one or glorifying another food as a cure for cancer or heart disease. A good example is olive oil. If you just dump it on a high-fat diet, its only effect will be to make you even fatter faster. But as part of the Mediterranean diet, olive oil is responsible for delivering a strong antioxidant load and changing your cholesterol in a very favorable way by increasing your good cholesterol.

So which diet is best? The best one delivers you into old age in good health without disability, while steering you around the major stumbling blocks, cancer and heart disease. Only then do you want to look at how lean the people are who eat these diets. Clearly if a diet has a high level of heart disease or cancer but leaves you rail thin, you'll be interested only if you want to be a good-looking corpse. The big loser from the outset is the American diet, with strikingly high levels of breast cancer, prostate cancer, colon cancer, and heart disease . . . even if eaten in quantities small enough to stay thin. The contest is then among the diet of Crete, the Asian diet, and the Sonoran diet. This chapter will outline the general benefits of all three and how they utilize the principles of this book by making your brain feel good, killing your hunger, and cutting your insulin.

THE ASIAN DIET

Oldways Preservation & Exchange Trust, a nonprofit food and nutrition education organization based in Boston, gained international fame and recognition for advocating traditional diets from around the world to maintain health. Oldways presented the Cretan diet of 1960 as the epitome of a healthy diet. Since then, they struck out to identify other cultures that offer healthy, appetizing ways to eat. Their latest triumph is the Asian diet. It is based on observations and epidemiological studies of dietary patterns — in South and East Asia including China, Japan, South Korea, India, Thailand, Vietnam, Cambodia, Indonesia, Malaysia, the Philippines, and other related Pacific Rim areas — linking nutrition and chronic disease patterns. There is no single country that nutritionists, research scientists, and epidemiologists have isolated as better than the others. They prefer to lump all these countries into one diet to combine the tremendous culinary wealth of all into one extended menu. While Korea appears to be the culture with the least body fat, it is China that has been studied the most extensively.

BENEFITS

T. Colin Campbell, Ph.D., chief investigator of the China-Cornell-Oxford Project on Nutrition at Cornell University in Ithaca, New York, is convinced that leanness is directly related to the composition of the diet. "People on a plant-based diet that is low in fat, low in animal protein, and high in fiber can afford to consume more calories because the foods burn off the calories as body heat."

Low fat

Only 14 percent of China's calories come from fat, compared to about 34 percent in the U.S. The Chinese average only 34 grams of fat a day.

Very high fiber

The Chinese average 77 grams of fiber a day, contrasted to only 10 grams in the U.S.

Low glucose load

The proper Chinese diet is also a low glucose load diet. Ironically, in 1974 both the developed and the developing world ate roughly the same amount of carbohydrates, 1,680 calories per day, but the kind of carbohydrates were strikingly different. In the developing world, 98 percent of the carbos came from cereals, roots, and other staples. In the developed world, 62 percent came from those foods, the rest came from fruits and sugars. The developing world ate hard carbos while we ate fast-burning carbos. Americans added to this carbohydrate load lots of extra fat calories of the worst kind: saturated fats and hydrogenated fats.

Leanness

Anthropologist Stephen Bailey, Ph.D., of Tufts says, "In terms of populations that are clearly well nourished, where there's no evidence of famine, I would say Korea and Japan are the leanest, based on height, weight, and skinfold measurements."

Health

The Japanese, in the most recent World Health Organization survey, had the world's highest life expectancy for both men and women coupled with the lowest rate of coronary artery disease and breast cancer for women. Where the Asian diet falls down is in the area of cancer, where it has a higher rate than Greece, the gold standard, but still lower than the U.S.

Longevity

Okinawa is home to the longest-lived people on earth. Local officials have kept records for over 115 years and can document that there are more centenarians in Okinawa, Japan, than anywhere else. Walk through the villages. You'll be struck that at eight or ninety-eight, everyone remains lean and taut. You'll see six generations all living together, with the oldest often the most active. They credit a spectacular diet rich in fish and "magic" fruits and vegetables that combine incredible taste with spectacular nutrition.

DISADVANTAGES

Asian foods are harder to shop for and cook than foods found in the Mediterranean diet, not because of their complexity, but because of our unfamiliarity with cooking them. The Asian diet is a much bigger change from a Western diet than is the Mediterranean. The major high-glycemic food is white rice, which can make weight loss difficult if eaten in high quantities.

THE ASIAN DIET PYRAMID

To combine all the nutritional assets of the Asian countries, Oldways established an Asian Diet Pyramid to serve as a what-to-eat guide. Recently released, it reflects the Asian dietary traditions historically associated with good health. Like the Mediterranean Diet Pyramid, the Asian Diet Pyramid challenges the adequacy of the USDA's Food Guide Pyramid. A chief complaint against the American Food Guide Pyramid made by experts in the fields of nutrition science and medicine has been the grouping of meat, poultry, and eggs with plant sources such as nuts and legumes in the "meat group." The Mediterranean and Asian Pyramids carefully distinguish between animal and plant foods. The pyramid is as follows: The base is made of rice, rice products, noodles, breads, millet, corn, and other grains, which are minimally refined. For the purposes of this book, you want to stick with starches that have a low glucose load and are high in fiber. There should be a narrow base to this triangle to avoid overeating grains that can make you fat. The middle is divided among fruits, legumes, nuts and seeds, and vegetables. For the purposes of this book, you want to pick most of your foods from this group. The top is divided between daily vegetable oils, optional daily fish, shellfish, or dairy (dairy is not usually part of the healthy Asian diet except in India), weekly eggs and poultry, weekly sweets, and monthly meat. Sake, wine, beer, other alcoholic beverages, and tea are written next to the pyramid, indicating low to moderate use.

Plant food is the core of the daily intake in the traditional Asian diets. Common plant foods include rice and other grains, noodles, flatbreads, potatoes, fruits, vegetables (including sea vegetables), nuts, seeds, beans, various soy foods, other legumes, vegetable and nut oils, herbs and spices, and plant-based beverages including tea, wine, and beer. When eaten in sufficient amounts, this healthy Asian diet provides all of the known essential vitamins, minerals, and fiber that promote health. This healthy diet is low in both saturated and total fat, but according to Oldways, future research is needed to clarify the impacts of the highly saturated coconut and palm oils that are used in some cultures.

Meat is used for flavor, not as the core of the meal, so that consumption is small. The most interesting shortfall of meat, even for low-fat varieties, is that it is a fiber-free, antioxidant-free food. Contrast that with beans, which are rich in minerals, vitamins, calcium, fiber, and antioxidants. A high consumption of fatty meats is associated with a higher incidence of chronic disease. (A recent study linked non-Hodgkins lymphoma to a high-fat red meat diet in women.) Dr. T. Colin Campbell has shown that when rats are fed a 20 percent protein diet, it turns on tumor growth. The growth is stopped by decreasing the protein intake to 6 percent.

Japan and other Asian countries consume wine, beer, and other alcoholic beverages, which in moderation or at meals may act in a favorable way in blood fats, as wine does in the Mediterranean diet.

For terrific suggestions on how to develop an Asian meal plan, I suggest the following books:

ASIAN
Terrific Pacific Cookbook, by Anya von Bremzen (Workman)
Beyond Bok Choy, by Rosa Lo San Ross (Artisan/Workman)
China Express, by Nina Simonds (William Morrow)
Classic Chinese Cuisine, by Nina Simonds (Chapters Publishers &
    Booksellers)

THE CRETAN DIET: THE PREMIER
MEDITERRANEAN DIET
The Rockefeller Foundation undertook a study in 1948 on the island of Crete to explore the diet of an "underdeveloped country," which showed that adults living in regions bordering the Mediterranean Sea showed some of the lowest rates of chronic disease in the world and had life expectancy among the highest. The effects were not linked to

educational level, socioeconomic status, or health care expenditure. There are sixteen countries bordering the Mediterranean, but it was Ancel Keys's work on the Greek island of Crete that represents the epitome of the healthy Mediterranean diet.

BENEFITS
Low saturated fat
High fiber
Low glucose load
The Mediterranean diet has been mistaken as the pasta diet. In Crete, not a lot of pasta is eaten, and the overall glucose load has dropped enormously because olive oil is substituted for carbohydrates in a big way. How much? According to Oldways Preservation & Trust, the Mediterranean diet is about 30 percent fat. Annie Copps of Oldways says, "It's even healthy at as high as 40 percent if the person is active and the fat is mostly vegetarian based."

Leanness
The Cretans of 1960 were indeed lean and fit. The big jump in fat in-take and calories has widened their girth.

Health
Oldways and the Harvard School of Public Health both point to the Mediterranean diet, Cretan edition, circa 1960, as the healthiest diet documented in recent history, since it could boast the lowest inci-dence of coronary artery disease and of cancer. Greeks still do very well today. The Greeks, in the most recent World Health Organiza-tion survey, have the second highest life expectancy for both men and women (77.5 and 81.7 years, respectively) coupled with the lowest rate of cancers. (See the Appendix for a complete comparison.) But they have lost the heart disease edge to the Japanese. What changed? Greece has nearly doubled its animal fat, potato, and egg intake while quadrupling the amount of meat. Where the traditional Cretan diet was virtually all vegetarian, it is now becoming far higher in meat.

ADVANTAGES

The big advantage of the Cretan diet over the Asian diet is that all of the foods are readily available at stores in virtually every community in America. They are foods we are used to eating.

THE GREEK FOODS, CIRCA 1960

The Greeks can thank Pythagoras for their good health. He introduced vegetarianism and abstinence from meat into Greece in the sixth to fifth centuries B.C. The diet of 1960 was low in saturated fat. Dr. Ancel Keys concluded that the culprits in countries like the United States are saturated fatty acids from the fat of meat and dairy products. The average American diet contains three to four times more beef, veal, pork, and chicken than the diets of Greece. Moreover, on the average, the Mediterranean meat is relatively lean compared to the meat consumed by Americans. In Crete, the fat that is present is mostly in the form of olive oil. The Cretan diet is high in complex carbohydrates from grains and legumes, and high in fiber from vegetables and fruit. Fresh plants, cereals, and olive oil secure a high intake of B carotene, vitamin C, tocopherols, and minerals. The diet is filled with olive oil, leaves from lettuce, spinach, Swiss chard, pasta, purslane, and many different kinds of vegetables, cheese, fruit, and wine. Why, with the current pasta witch-hunt, is pasta allowed in the diet? The preponderance of slow-burning carbos and fats reduces the overall glycemic load to a very low level.

Olive Oil

The Cretan diet was high in total fat but low in saturated fatty acids thanks to the olive oil. The Greeks had a big leg up on the rest of us because olives may have first been cultivated in Crete. Greek Orthodox priests even anoint babies with olive oil at their christenings. How good is olive oil? In his article "Diet and Health: What Should We Eat?" Walter Willett of the Harvard School of Public Health proposed that it is olive oil, not extremely low-fat diets, that may be the reason for good health. Can the diet of Crete work for a Western industrialized country? Over six hundred French patients, all recovering from heart attacks, participated in a randomized, prospective prevention trial. The study compared an adaptation to the Cretan diet with the usual prescribed heart healthy diet. After a follow-up period of 27 months, all cardiovascular events, including recurrent heart attack and death, were significantly decreased by fully 70 percent in the group consuming the Cretan diet. In adapting the diet, doctors realized it was impossible to impose olive oil as the only edible fat, so they selected canola oil as the fat most like olive oil in its fatty acid composition. If you use canola oil, make sure that it's not hydrogenated.

MEDITERRANEAN MEALS

Both the Cretan and Puglian meals were prepared by nationally known food writer and author of *The Mediterranean Diet Cookbook*, Nancy Harmon Jenkins. Puglia is an area in Italy located in the most eastern part of the country, at the heel of the boot. It is where the data for a great number of the early studies on the Mediterranean diet were gathered.

Cretan Day

Breakfast: Dense, grainy, coarse bread, toasted or not; low- or nonfat yogurt

Snack: Fruit

Lunch: A light vegetable soup (tomatoes, onions, bulgur wheat); a small piece of grilled fish with olive oil; a green salad with a little feta cheese and olives, dressed with oil and lemon juice; coarse bread, fresh seasonal fruit; a glass of white wine; a minicup of black coffee

Dinner: Seasonal vegetables (e.g., in summer, tomatoes, peppers, eggplant; in winter, beans, chickpeas, wheatberries or lentils, potatoes), stewed together with garlic and onions in olive oil; coarse bread; a hard cheese like kefalotiri, a glass of red wine; a cup of coffee or herbal chamomile or mint tea

Puglian Day

Breakfast: Toasted dense, grainy, coarse bread, toasted with a little olive oil and some fresh cheese or maybe chopped greens left over from supper the night before

Snack: Fruit

Lunch: Hard-wheat pasta (no egg) with bitter greens (broccoli rabe); fish stew (mussels, shrimp, monkfish, cooked with tomatoes, onion, garlic); bread made with semolina flour; green salad of lettuces, dressed with oil and vinegar; a glass of white wine; sopratavola (a plain raw vegetable like fennel), celery, chicory, served at the end of the meal to clear the palate; orange, cherries, peaches, or figs for dessert

Dinner: Frittata omelette made with a mixture of whole eggs and egg whites, fresh mint, and onions; small coarse bread rolls, called *friselle,* piled with chopped tomatoes, arugula, and an oil and vinegar dressing; a glass of red wine; a handful of green almonds and a few cherries with honey for dessert

"The Mediterranean diet is so obviously healthy. It is full of fresh vegetables, is high in fiber and very low in saturated fat. The next best thing is that these foods are familiar to us. It doesn't require us to make great leaps to enjoy the tradition," says Nancy.

THE SONORAN DIET

If you're looking for a really simple diet with spectacular results this is it. It's my favorite by far and easy to eat. I came across the Sonoran diet, named for the northwestern province of Mexico, during a trip to visit the Pima Indians. I was so struck by their remarkable vitality, good humor, and leanness that I vowed to try it. In a small cafe in the town of Maicoba, which is about six hours by switchback road from running water and electricity, deep in the Sierra Madre, I had my first Sonoran feast. The core is made from beans and corn tortillas. These two simple foods deliver 95 percent of your nutrients and tremendous filling power. This is the diet that the Pima eat to grow to over one hundred years of age with boundless vigor. The whole family cooked. They baked the corn tortillas from scratch. The pinto beans were boiled, then crushed into a coarse paste and heated in a skillet with a small amount of vegetable oil. This is served with a mixed vegetable dish and peaches for dessert. This makes a delicious, filling, and invigorating meal.

BENEFITS

High soluble fiber

I've come across no diet with a higher amount of soluble fiber, as much as 35 grams a day. This is an incredible dose, one that assures a very even blood sugar level and long-lasting satiety.

High total fiber

The Pima eat a minimum of 50 grams and some up to 100 grams. Even big-city dwellers get at least 35 grams a day.

Prolonged energy

Beans give you a super-low release for as long as eight hours. After a simple bean tortilla lunch, I wasn't hungry until bedtime, even after a two-hour moonlight bike ride through the mountains.

Low glucose load

The overall glucose load is stunningly low even for a high-carbo diet. Beans weigh in at 15; the tortillas, at 38.

Makes your brain feel good

Simple but highly effective means of making brain chemicals. The heavy concentration of tyrosine in the beans acts to make you alert from dawn into the evening. Lowering the bean intake in the evening and adding carbos in the form of potatoes makes more serotonin to ensure sleep.

OUTCOME

Oldways is just beginning to look at Latin and South American diets for their health effects. What we do know is that the Mexican Pima do extraordinarily well on it. With a genetic predisposition to diabetes, in reality they suffer less diabetes than the Mexican population as a whole. With an incredible risk for overwhelming obesity, they remain thin on these foods. Some will say they are lean because of their hard physical labor, but I believe that fitness is possible only because of the energizing effects of their diet.

Leanness

We also know that billions of other people around the world remain taut and trim on bean grain diets. On a visit last year to the Acuapa in Nicaragua, I was struck by the lean, muscular fitness of the people. You look at young men's washboard abdomens covered with nearly paper-thin folds of flesh rather than rolls of fat. Their diet is simple: red beans (they don't like darker ones), rice, plantains, tortillas, cabbage salads, and papayas. Twice a week they eat meat, either chicken or beef. Do they have any dietary deficiencies? Yes, they are low on vitamin A and iron, which can easily be made up for by spinach, pumpkin, carrots, and cantaloupe, and dark green, leafy vegetables, respectively.

WHERE YOU CAN GO WRONG

Just before leaving for Mexico, I stopped at a Mexican restaurant in Los Angeles and ordered "super-healthy beans and rice." The beans were refried and packed with fat. I asked why and was told, "If we don't put in the fat, we can't sell the stuff." Yet in Mexico, most Americans are surprised by how much better the meal tastes than the fat-laden U.S. version.

SAMPLE DAY

Here's the stripped-down basic diet eaten by subsistence farmers:

> *Breakfast:* Flour tortillas, beans
> *Lunch:* Corn tortillas, beans, mixed vegetables
> *Dinner:* Corn tortillas, potatoes, peaches

Here's a more robust version of the Sonoran diet prepared by Arline D. Salbe, Ph.D., R.D., the research nutritionist for the National Institutes of Health, National Institute of Diabetes and Digestive and Kidney Diseases, Clinical Diabetes and Nutrition Section in Phoenix, Arizona.

> *Breakfast:* Whole wheat burrito stuffed with three cooked egg whites and chopped green chilies, wrapped in a whole wheat fat-free tortilla; plain fat-free yogurt with fresh strawberries

Lunch: Fish tacos made with freshly grilled tuna chunks, shredded romaine lettuce, chopped fresh tomato, shredded cabbage all topped with a spicy low-fat dressing (salsa, no-fat yogurt, low- or no-fat mayo, pickle relish); fresh fruit

Snack: Fat-free baked tortilla chips with carrot, celery, and jicama slices

Dinner: Chicken fajitas: white meat chicken marinated and grilled along with onions, red and green sweet peppers, and tomato chunks, wrapped in a whole wheat fat-free tortilla, served with steamed brown rice, cooked black beans, and pico de gallo (fresh tomato salsa) sauce

Says Arline, "This is wonderful cuisine for providing low-fat, high-fiber foods with zesty great taste. It's light, easy to prepare, and fun to eat. Foods don't have to contain lard, lots of meat, or lots of spices to be delicacies. This can really put the spark in a routine diet."

part four *Fat-Loss Accelerators*

Fat-Ripping Exercises

If you're like most Americans and don't exercise regularly, at this point in the book you are saying to yourself: "Oh God, here he goes. He's going to sell me an exercise program. I'm going to have to ply the predawn darkness powerwalking at the local mall . . . forget it!" I'm *not* going to try to convince you. Honest! However, hear me out! The reason you and most Americans don't exercise regularly is because you can't. You just don't have the energy, the strength, the brain power, or internal motivation to exercise. With what you've learned so far in this book, you can dramatically change the way your body operates so that you'll barely be able to contain your glee each time you have the opportunity to exercise. When you feel that happening, come back to this chapter for the best and most entertaining fat-ripping exercises there are.

Conventional Wisdom
Power stroll at the mall, reload those carbos at each and every shop.

LEAN
Intense! Blade, bike, climb.

ROAD MAP
This chapter outlines the sports that burn the most calories either because you can exercise vigorously easily to burn many calories in a short time or you can exercise for long periods without exhaustion or soreness. It also critiques the sports that don't burn many calories and may not help you with weight loss. At the end of the chapter are pointers on how to train smart.

BENEFITS

NO NEED TO DIET

Tufts anthropologist Stephen Bailey, Ph.D., recently returned from a month in Tibet. His observation? "The more I look at things, the more I realize that physical activity is as important as what people eat. I was looking at Tibetans who were eating massive amounts of yak butter and saturated fat and doing just fine. It's because they are so active that they burn the fat before it can be deposited in their arteries."

DUMPS THE WORST KIND OF FAT

Jack Wilmore, Ph.D., professor of kinesiology and health education at the University of Texas at Austin, has researched the health benefits of exercise for years. He says, "Our whole focus has been on the role of exercise. Physical inactivity is a big player in the chronic diseases including obesity." A research study in progress in Dr. Wilmore's lab shows exercise alone (with no change in diet) has a positive effect on belly fat.

BEST PREDICTOR OF SUCCESS

Long-term weight-loss studies from the NIH started out with suppositions of the importance of psychological factors such as willpower, knowledge, and commitment to weight loss. They found that the most consistent predictor of long-term success is exercise level.

GENERATES HUNGER FOR FOODS THAT MAKE YOU LEAN

If you're having a difficult time giving up fats, listen to this. William McCarthy, Ph.D., director of Science at the Pritikin Longevity Center in Santa Monica, California, says, "When the body expends calories in exercise it engenders hunger for carbohydrate. The body has no interest in fat but in carbohydrate. I'm beginning to think that Americans are not eating enough fruits and vegetables because they're not exercising enough to engender the hunger for the carbohydrate required."

SPEEDS WEIGHT LOSS

Exercise offers startling advantages for weight loss. Xavier Pi-Sunyer, of St. Luke's Hospital in New York City, studied groups of fat and thin people. Both groups began exercise programs and both increased the calories that they burned considerably. However, overweight people didn't eat more to match the amount they expended. You'll be surprised at how fast exercise speeds weight loss when you don't make up for the calories that you expend in exercise. This chapter will help you find the most effective and highest calorie-burning machines and exercise routines for you.

Here are some additional benefits from the latest research on exercise:

- Increases the overall size of the deficit between calories eaten and calories expended
- Facilitates mobilization of fat from fat cells, especially those around the belly that are hardest to get at
- Increases the loss of body fat while preserving muscle
- Blunts the drop in resting metabolism that frequently accompanies weight loss by preserving muscle mass

BETTER WEAPONS, LEANER BODY

One big reason the fit are fit is that they have better weapons . . . awesomely better equipment than the also-rans: from 4000 PT StairMaster and titanium Light Speed mountain bikes to five-wheeled, carbon-fiber Bont in-line speed blades. There is a persnickety attitude in the public health community that exercise must be universally available. So what you will hear them recommend are walking to the bus, climbing a flight of stairs, or pulling weeds in the garden. Talk about defenseless against the rising tide of obesity. It's like a Muslim walking through Serbia unarmed. To rip off the fat, choose the best weapons you can afford. They allow you to burn off far more calories for far less effort . . . but more important, they make exercise play.

OVERRATED EXERCISES

Many popularly advocated exercises have little potential to burn large numbers of calories without an extremely dedicated long-term training program. Here are some examples.

SWIMMING

For any distance longer than a hundred yards, the major muscles of the lower body get very little exercise. In a long-distance crawl, they are used more for balance than propulsion. Most of us will simply never develop the aerobic ability in our upper body muscles to burn very many calories. A top swimmer can turn over a mile in 16 minutes, the very fit in 30 minutes, quite fit in 45 minutes, and the rest of us an hour or more. At the slower paces, frighteningly few calories are burned. Some studies even show weight gain during a swimming program of exercise. If you're fast, stick with it; if you float, get out.

AEROBIC DANCE

Aerobics are so hard on the body that up to 50 percent of instructors have been injured on the job. Total calorie burn is paltry, and muscle-building potential is meager. Aerobic instructors may look great, but sneak a peek to see how much time they pump iron.

STROLLING

Walking is widely promoted as the number-one exercise in America. But unless you are a racewalker, you're not burning huge numbers of calories. Where an Olympian can walk a 6½-minute mile, faster than many marathoners, most modern power walkers are lucky to hit 18 minutes a mile. Simple walking does have a very profound effect on the physiology of obesity, it does decrease insulin levels, shift blood sugar into muscle and away from fat, and it will get your metabolism going, but it's not a fat ripper unless you really push the envelope or put in really big mileage.

EXERCISE BIKE

Many exercise bikes are constructed to discourage exercise. Since the maximum effort required is when the pedals are in the 12 and 6 o'clock position instead of the 9 and 3, you are at a tremendous mechanical disadvantage. Even top road cyclists have a hard time adjusting to a modestly priced exercise bike. Recent studies show only a modest calorie expenditure even on a good one.

CROSS-COUNTRY SKI MACHINES

This machine does distribute the load of exercise over all the major groups. I've owned a NordicTrack, but found that it's hard to get enough intensity to burn large numbers of calories. That's because it's hard to turn up the resistance high enough to work out the legs, while the friction drum for the upper body workout gets too hard too fast and gives an uncomfortable grating sensation like fingernails across a chalkboard. However, roller skiing is another matter. This is a terrific calorie burner that you can undertake even if you live in Brazil. You wear conventional cross-country ski boots, which are attached with a binding to a roughly two-foot "ski" with wheels at either end. The wheels have a rachet system that allows you to push off without going backward. The poles have tips that are hard enough and sharp enough to stick into the pavement. There's even a new fully suspended dirt road variety.

HEALTH RIDERS

These machines too are hard to ride long enough to burn the calories you need to lose weight.

FAT-RIPPING EXERCISES

What does work? Exercises that use large groups of muscles with minimal strain on any ligaments, bones, and joints. The more muscles that are used, the greater the number of calories burned, the lower the perceived exertion, the longer and harder you can exercise. The best fat-ripping exercise allows you to burn a lot of calories in a short period of time or are easy enough on the body to burn many calories over a long time.

Penn State's Dr. Bill Evans says, "Because the larger the muscle group that you use, the greater calorie expenditure, you want to run, cross-country ski, cycle, or do any exercise that uses the large muscle groups, which will burn lots of calories. The higher the intensity of the exercise, the greater number of calories you will use." Exercise has gotten a bad reputation because it appears painful to casual observers. But look at a top cyclist in training. There's not even a grimace. The better you get, the less exertion you perceive at any given level of exercise. When you begin, every motion seems painful. There's a reason you feel pain: Your body is telling you to take it easy. Let your body accommodate to the strain you're putting on it. If you're not shooting for the Olympics, there's never a need to suffer serious discomfort when you exercise. Just pay attention to your perceived exertion. Rate your workouts. Back off when it hurts. Give yourself several days of slow workouts. When you go hard, it should be because your muscles feel restless, itching — even anxious — to get a great workout.

Here's what really works:

HIKING AND BIKING

I asked Mark Black of the famed Canyon Ranch which exercises they found unfit people could take up with ease to burn a maximum number of calories. He recommended two strongly: hiking and biking. "Both of these sports are excellent for people who want to lose weight, because they are examples of intense caloric expenditures of energy. We have a lot of beginners, and believe it or not people tend to go longer on the bike or hiking because the scenery is like entertainment." Neither is monotonous, like so many indoor activities. "These sports are more enjoyable because there's a recreational edge to them as opposed to just a clinical workout." While many become bored before they can get the right amount of an activity to lose weight, these sports are easier to get to a fat-burning level. "People end up wanting to go longer than they ever thought they would."

These sports are also great because they're safe. Mark adds, "As long as there are no outstanding, preexisting conditions, these exercises are really safe. You would think it would be hard on the body, but it strengthens your body. The bike is hard on the butt but that's all. These are user-friendly sports. They become strangely addictive."

There's also a great deal of freedom. The nature of the activities are such that you can cut back, speed up, or stop and have a drink of water.

Rank beginners can try two hours of hiking or one to two hours of riding with a stop. Here's an individual look at each activity.

Hiking

This is the easiest and lowest tech of all fat-ripping exercises. It's the mainstay of many spa programs. No matter how overweight or out of shape you are, you can hike. Hiking burns massive numbers of calories. What's more, as they found over the years at Canyon Ranch, even the first day out you can put in an hour or more. That's not true of almost any other exercise. You don't need a mountain to hike, just undulating terrain, like a golf course. With proper technique, there is no pounding of your joints. Lifting your body uphill expends a huge number of calories. Carefully lowering your body works the hamstrings for a good calorie burn on the descent.

Equipment: The proper footwear is vital. You'll need traction and ankle support. You should have a roomy toe box, so the boot should probably be one half size larger than your normal shoe size to avoid blisters, since your feet will expand. Your socks should be thicker so when you go downhill your foot won't slide forward in the boot and jam into the front of the boot as it will without thick socks. If you hate the big clunky boots, the new high-tech hiking sneakers are a dream. They're light and fast, like running shoes, with a great, grippy sole and lots of ankle protection. Called "approach" shoes, you can find them at good camping stores. I bought the Nike trail-running shoe. It's the single most comfortable shoe I've ever owned and even feels like I'm being propelled up the trail.

If you're going to be hiking in cool or cold weather, knowing the layering system is invaluable because it allows you to adjust to changing conditions: wet, dry, hot, or cold extremes. In the desert, temperature swings can be forty degrees from morning to night. Your first layer should be a synthetic material like polypropylene or Capelene, which will wick moisture away from your body so you stay dry. Cotton stays wet and doesn't dry, which makes it okay for high temperatures but not for cool ones. Your second layer is your insulating layer, which will keep you warm. Choose fabrics like pile or a cotton sweat shirt. Your third layer is your shell, which will hold that heat in. Don't forget a baseball-type hat for sun protection. Remember the Scandinavian expression: "There's no such thing as cold weather, just cold clothing."

Water: Don't let yourself go too long without water. Canyon Ranch hikers drink at least two quarts of water on each hike. Use a sports drink to increase the amount you'll want to drink. The Camelback, a mini backpack-style fluid carrier, is a great way to carry the fluid without having to fumble with canteens or water bottles.

Cell phone: Make sure someone knows where you will be and when you'll be back. If you have access to or own a cellular phone, it will probably be the single most important piece of safety gear you can carry. Lives have been saved with them.

Biking

OK, call me fatso. After a long hard winter there's an extra ten pounds registering on the scale. I never worry about it because I know I can ride unlimited distances on a bike and rip the fat off within a month. Bikes perfectly accommodate to any frame or size and to most orthopedic injuries. Where it would take years of preparation to run a marathon, you could ride a 50-mile bike race within weeks of beginning. I love mountain bikes because of the tremendous comfort level. Mine has a twin suspension system for an extremely pleasing ride. This is an intense whole-body workout once you get off the road and up some hills. It's easy on your back and your body.

Be careful not to buy a bike that is too cheap. Those bikes build up so much resistance at low speed that you can't exercise very hard. The better the bike, the better the workout. They're the ultimate time machine, since you can ride at very competitive speeds to a very old age. They'll keep your legs springy, elastic, and powerful.

Buy bike shorts with a padded crotch to avoid saddle discomfort. Also important are helmets, and gloves — to avoid blisters and to get a better grip on the bike.

SPINNING

So, old-fashioned indoor exercise bikes don't get much respect on the weight-loss front, but that's largely a motivational problem. For those who love the motivation, the music, the electricity and sense of companionship that can come with aerobic dance classes — but who simply can't risk the high-impact pounding or the embarrassment of appearing uncoordinated — there is something new in clubs across the U.S. and in thirty countries around the world. It's called spinning and it's done in a class setting, on a new kind of stationary bike — one that allows a dynamic cardiovascular workout.

You stand on the pedals to climb imaginary steep hills, and change hand positions as the "terrain" shifts. You'll hear all different kinds of music, not just the disco beat of aerobics classes but everything from show tunes to New Age music to rock and roll. You don't have to worry about choreography, looking like a great dancer, or following a routine with which you're unfamiliar. This is an intense cardiovascular-training and mental-strengthening workout.

Equipment: Spinning creator Johnny G., a martial arts black belt who cycled across America in 9.5 days, worked with the Schwinn bike company to develop the Johnny G. Spinner bike. You can buy it and use it in your home if you're motivated enough. Or you can find it in health clubs and freestanding spinning centers around the country. Reebok and other companies are putting out their version of both the bike and the training program, and it's red-hot.

Just how intense is the exercise? It peaks at 85 percent of your target heart rate, and then drops off periodically to recovery periods at 65 percent.

CROSS-COUNTRY SKIING

This is called the queen of aerobic sports because it burns the greatest number of calories per hour of any sport, hour after hour. I can burn a good 1,600 calories an hour. That means I've lost a pound of fat in a little over two hours. The fastest form of the sport is called skating and can be learned in a morning, using super-high-tech short skis called "revolutions" or "tempos." You can easily undertake a three-hour ski with little basic fitness. The time flies.

STAIR MACHINES

These allow you to lift your entire body weight with minimal strain on tendons, joints, or ligaments. You can start with very small steps then move up to a complete flexion and extension of the leg muscles as you get stronger. The more you weigh, the better the workout, so if you're overweight, expect to burn lots of calories. I burn 900 an hour at a very modest exercise load, and a heart rate of only 120. Since you lift your body weight each time you step, you are using the powerful muscles of your buttocks, thighs, and calves, and lower back. This burns double the number of calories as running but with far less strain. You can hammer a stair machine every day of the week.

Equipment: Be certain the machine you use has fully independent leg action so you don't endanger your knees. The StairMaster 4000 PT and ClimbMax by Tectrix Fitness Equipment of Irvine, California, are reliable machines. If you have a heavy frame, are nearing fifty, or are seriously overweight, make certain to use heavy-duty cross-training shoes with a custom foot bed. You'll find that without the foot bed, you stand a much higher chance of dropping the metatarsal heads (the end of the long bones in your foot), which can become painful and debilitating over time. Not that stair climbing is that high a foot stress — you'd want to do the same thing for hiking, running, walking, or any other pounding activity.

ROWING ERGOMETERS

These engage most major muscle groups to rip off fat. You can't maintain the intensity as long as in cross-country skiing, but the calorie burn is enormous. Most practiced oarsmen row in sets of 2,000 meters. Rowing machines simulate real rowing in a very modest fashion. However, the Concept II rowing ergometer has a very realistic rowing motion, is reasonably priced, and is a tremendous way to burn calories. I've kept one in the bedroom in front of the TV to watch the news at night with my one-year-old on my back.

ROLLER BLADING

Too old to roller blade? Santa Barbara's bike paths are loaded with sixty- and seventy-year-olds. This sport is very kind to your muscles and burns lots of calories. Be sure to learn good form so you get great leg extension. Just one or two lessons will get you on the way. With good form, your legs will bend through a complete range of motion starting with your thighs parallel to the ground and ending with your leg completely outstretched. The arm motion and upper-body activity bring all the major muscle groups into play. Go for 76 mm wheels for fast turnover. If your balance is good, get the low-cut racing boots.

TREADMILL

The *Journal of the American Medical Association* rated the treadmill as the number-one indoor exercise machine. Rather than running on them, I like to increase the elevation and power hike. For the occasional athlete, the treadmill burns the most calories of any indoor machine. Researchers at the Medical College of Wisconsin and the Veterans Affairs Medical Centre in Milwaukee found the treadmill burned off 40 percent more calories than other workout machines. The treadmill burned 700 calories an hour, compared to only 500 for the same level of exertion on a stationary bike. The treadmill machine was also compared to an Airdyne (a bike with an upper-body push-pull system), a cross-country ski simulator, a rowing ergometer, and a stairstep machine. The treadmill won because it inflicted the least pain at the highest intensity. The other machines caused much more hurt or pain at lower levels of exercise, limiting their effectiveness. Here's the catch: If you are a highly trained athlete who has mastered another machine such as the rowing ergometer or stair machine, you could burn many more calories because you've pushed the pain threshold to a very high level. However, if you're just starting to get fit, the treadmill will be easier for you to burn more calories.

LONG-DISTANCE RUNNING

True, you can burn a mountain of calories with this one, but it takes years of training to get to the volume and intensity needed to really burn calories. If you're rail thin with a light frame, narrow hips, and a perfect anatomy for running, good luck! If you're really overweight or have a heavy frame, pass this one up. You'll make little quick progress and spend years getting to the point you can burn as many calories as you can in the first week of cycling. If Bill Clinton had traded in jogging for blading or biking, he'd have put dozens of cartoonists out of work years ago.

A NOTE TO THOSE WHO ARE OVERWEIGHT

If you are overweight, you may be surprised to learn that you have a bigger muscle mass than an average individual who is of normal weight. But if you run, walk, or stroll you cannot use that to your advantage because you are carrying so much extra weight. Just as water neutralizes those extra pounds by buoying you up, any exercise equipment that supports your body weight allows you to work those bigger muscles with no disadvantage from your body-fat stores. Now if you take this a step further and use equipment that actually employs your biggest muscle groups to their maximal advantage, you will have true fat-ripping exercises, cycling and stair machines being the two standout examples. For weight training you have an even bigger running start, because an overweight person also has more muscle than a trim person.

A NOTE TO ATHLETES

If you already are an athlete, even an Olympian, you will be astounded to learn the truly massive amount of exercise you've needed to do for years to overcome the damage you do with dirt-poor nutrition. High glucose loads followed by high insulin spikes ruin workouts. I can't remember the number of workouts where I bonked and just plain stopped dead in my tracks from diet-induced light-headedness. One major reason that Barry Sears's Zone diet worked so well with the Stanford swim team is that he reduced their glucose load. A study from the University of Buffalo also showed that a higher fat diet that reduced glucose load improved performance. The higher fat diet may actually build more machinery, called mitochondria, in your cells to process oxygen. To improve your own performance substantially, reread the chapter on cutting glucose load and the fueling section of "Feedforward Eating."

HOW HARD TO EXERCISE
INTENSE EXERCISE

When you exercise at 80 percent or more of your capacity, you burn huge numbers of calories and kick your body's fat-burning metabolism into overdrive for hours after you're finished. Once you're fit and can handle a bigger workout, three fifteen-minute bursts of intense aerobic activity, in addition to your regular workout, can really spur weight loss. Intense exercise is also a great long-term investment. Only intense exercise increases your longevity, according to a long-term study of 17,300 Harvard alumni published in the *New England Journal of Medicine*. Those who did the most intense exercise lived the longest.

MODERATE EXERCISE

Moderate exercise may not get you to 120, but it can substantially decrease your chance of dying young. The Centers for Disease Control and Prevention estimates that 250,000 deaths could be avoided each year if every sedentary American spent thirty minutes a day walking, climbing stairs, or just walking around the house. Stanford epidemiologist Dr. Ralph Paffenbarger says, "Even moderate exercise can reduce the risk of coronary heart disease, stroke, diabetes, colon cancer and clinical depression, and it stands to reason that if you reduce these risks you would automatically increase survival rates." Activities like walking and climbing stairs and sports, which burn 2,000 or more calories a week, lower death rates by one-quarter to one-third over the least active. It's also clear that even the most basic exercise has a substantial effect on fat by shifting dietary fat and carbohydrates away from fat and into muscle. It's the most important single metabolic function that exercise plays. That's given rise to the idea that there is an ideal fat-burning zone for exercise. Don't be fooled; the more you burn the more you lose, either by exercising longer or harder.

WEIGHT-LOSS INTENSITY

You really want whatever intensity you can sustain for a long period of time. Mark Black of Canyon Ranch says, "That's why I recommend that people never follow their friend who is super-fit and try to keep up with them. I see that all the time, and people inevitably end up saying, 'It's all over, hiking (or biking) sucks.' " As you get better, your intensity will increase. The reason I'm so keen on fat-ripping exercises is that many muscle groups doing moderate activity add up to an intense exercise for the body that's pain-free. It's this kind of activity that peels away the pounds without the need to count calories, although you'll still want to mine the medicinal powers of foods to boost your performance. For the last several years the popular press has written a great deal about low-intensity workouts. The conventional wisdom is that they are better for you because they burn more fat. Now here are the facts. Sure, you'll burn more fat than carbohydrates at a very low intensity. So if you're walking and burning 200 calories an hour, over half will be fat, or roughly 100 calories. But if you were exercising at a rate expending 1,600 calories an hour, you might burn 700 calories of fat.

CALORIE TABLES

Here's a look at how many calories you can burn in a variety of sports for selected weights. They can be deceptive since you may not be fit enough to exercise at the intensity indicated. The first table shows the incredible numbers of calories that men and women can burn when they are very, very good at a sport. That generally means years of conditioning.

That's why you want to get good at a sport where you know you can maintain a high intensity over a long time. The second chart shows a more reasonable calorie burn for men and women with only a modest level of fitness.

TRAINING SMART

As you get better and better at the sport you've chosen, you'll burn double or even triple the calories of your beginning level. If you're committed to that kind of effort, here's how to train most efficiently.

CROSS TRAINING

Two close complementary sports that use similar muscles are a great way to reduce the stress of overtraining and the risk of injury. I like

Calories Burned per Hour for Very Fit Men and Women

Activity	Men (180 lbs.)	Men (200 lbs.)	Women (130 lbs.)	Women (150 lbs.)
Cross-country skiing uphill	1,350	1,500	975	1,125
Cycling at 20 m.p.h.	1,309	1,455	945	1,091
Competitive speed skating	1,227	1,364	886	1,023
Rowing ergometer, very vigorously (200 watts)	982	1,091	709	818
Boxing, in ring	982	1,091	709	818
Handball	982	1,091	709	818
Rope jumping, fast	982	1,091	709	818
Squash	982	1,091	709	818
Kayaking	982	1,091	709	818
Running at 7 m.p.h.	941	1,045	680	784
Rock climbing, ascending rock	900	1,000	650	750
Swimming, crawl, fast	900	1,000	650	750
Bicycling, stationary, very vigorously (200 watts)	859	955	620	716

Calories Burned per Hour for Unfit to Modestly Fit Men and Women

Activity	Men (180 lbs.)	Men (200 lbs.)	Women (130 lbs.)	Women (150 lbs.)
Cross-country skiing at 5 to 8 m.p.h.	736	818	532	614
Mountain biking	695	773	502	580
Rowing machine	695	773	502	580
Moderate cycling	655	727	473	545
Running at 5 m.p.h.	655	727	473	545
Basketball game	655	727	473	545
Singles tennis	655	727	473	545
Swimming, crawl, slow	655	727	473	545
Snowshoeing	655	727	473	545
Stationary bike at moderate effort	573	636	414	477
Aerobics, high impact	573	636	414	477
Jogging	573	636	414	477
Hiking uphill	573	636	414	477
Brisk walking	491	545	355	409
Golf	368	409	266	307
Walking, 20-minute mile	245	273	177	205

Table adapted with permission from the American College of Sports Medicine, from *Med. Sci. Sports Experiments,* vol. 25, no. 1 (1993), pp. 71–80.

pairing roller blading with cycling, blading with cross-country skiing, or cycling with stair machines. Just when you start to feel stale in one sport, spend a day doing the other. You'll sharply reduce the amount of overuse while maintaining a very high level of conditioning.

INCREASING THE ANAEROBIC THRESHOLD

The preceding calorie chart above shows some outrageously high-calorie expenditures. The only way you can get close to those levels for a long period of time is by increasing the intensity to a point where your body begins to produce lactic acid. We called this the anaerobic threshold (AT), because faster speeds would drive major muscle groups to make enormous amounts of harmful lactic acid. Once you begin to produce lactic acid, you'll have to cut your pace. By increasing your AT, you can go faster in any endurance activity. Moving the AT should be the first and major speed goal of any endurance training program. Thirty to forty-five minutes of near-race-pace training once or twice a week is the most commonly used routine. When you are beginning a sport, natural intervals are the best way to move the AT, since you won't be able to maintain race pace for any significant length of time. That means brief periods of high intensity during a long moderately paced workout. The easiest way to do that is to pick up the pace on the crests of hills, then ease up on the way down. Since the body can adapt only if it has a chance to rest, train hard one day followed by two easy days. It's the surest way to become as fast as you can and recover the best you can.

There is no good self-administered test, but you can get a good sense of where your anaerobic threshold is by determining what your best pace is for thirty minutes. You'll find that the threshold occurs around the point where you have a nice heavily winded sensation but are short of air hunger. It's just past the point where you can carry on any kind of conversation. Once you pass over the threshold, you'll quickly build up too much lactic acid and be forced to slow or stop. Use your heart rate monitor to mark your pace. You'll quickly get a sense of the highest continuous heart rate you can maintain. Dr. William Kraemer, director of research at the Center for Sports Medicine at Penn State University, explains why the AT is so critical:

"The value of knowing about anaerobic threshold is that as athletes get in better and better shape, they can go harder and harder without running into excessive production of lactic acid. Your absolute maximum doesn't have to change at all. But if you push from 55 to 75 percent or 75 to 85 percent where you start really producing a lot of lactic acid, you're getting really fit."

HEART RATE MONITORS

I'm a big believer in heart rate monitors. You'll have no idea how hard you're training without a heart rate monitor. By using one, you can dramatically increase the number of calories you burn. That's because you'll easily be able to find the zone where you are burning the most calories. Without one, most Americans underexercise to an amazing degree. Where a heart rate of 160 might burn 1,400 calories an hour, I've found many friends barely hitting 100. They just don't know any better until they see the readout on a heart rate monitor. You wouldn't drive a car without a speedometer, and you shouldn't train without a heart rate monitor. They're pretty inexpensive now, many below $100. I bought a Polar Vantage, made by Polar Electo Inc., because I can download the results into my computer. I wear it as a wristwatch, then put the chestband on for exercise. Here's the table that shows the general range for heart rate.

- 100 percent is pretty hard to hit and impossible to maintain for more than a minute or two.
- 90 percent is what really top athletes can maintain on race day.
- 80 percent is what you'll want to hit on your one or two hard days a week, once you're in really good condition.

Heart Rate

Age	20	30	40	50	60	70	80	90
100%	200	190	180	170	160	150	140	130
90%	180	171	162	153	144	135	126	117
80%	160	152	144	136	128	120	112	104
70%	140	133	126	119	112	105	98	91
60%	120	114	108	102	96	90	84	78
50%	100	95	90	85	80	75	70	65
40%	80	76	72	68	64	60	56	52

- 70 percent is the practical top end for general fitness.
- 60 percent is what you need to hit for a good workout.
- Below 50 percent, you're coasting.

Get a sense of what your heart rate is at specific speeds in your sport. It really allows you to compete with yourself. When the monitor ticks the top of the scale, you know you're doing your best.

GETTING PSYCHED

Don't pick a sport for some pedestrian reason; see yourself as a sports hero and then choose an insanely great sport. Go crazy. Get fired up: Buy the magazines, visit all the Web sites, take a sports vacation, buy the greatest equipment.

Building a Fat-Burning Engine

Sitting at idle on a runway, a small executive jet can burn twenty gallons of fuel a minute. Its huge, powerful engines devour fuel even at rest. Like that jet, the more muscle you have, the more fuel you'll burn, even at rest. Although body building is an enormous time commitment, which is off-limits to most busy Americans, building a big muscular fuel-burning engine is not. Where body builders must hone every last fiber of muscle into sculptured perfection, you need only pump up your biggest muscle groups. These are easy to build with just a very few exercises that can be done at the gym, on the road, at work, or at home. The chest, buttock, thigh, back, and upper arm muscles develop quickly because they have the most genetic potential to grow. Even if you're the hardest of hard gainers, you can still build the muscle you need to have an engine that purrs like a lion. Fear not that you'll look like a musclehead, most people won't sprout geeky "Popeye" muscles without years of professional training. The more muscle mass you have, the more fuel you burn. Remember, as a woman, you'll lose four pounds of muscle mass every decade after forty. As a man, you'll lose six pounds per decade. To prevent the inexorable weight gain most of us experience in middle age, both men and women need to pump iron!

Conventional Wisdom
Muscles inevitably turn to fat.

LEAN
New muscle, no fat.

ROAD MAP

This chapter has the best exercises to build the most muscle in the shortest period. You will find only those muscles included that are large enough to burn many calories and yet are easy enough to make bigger quickly. Women over thirty need not be concerned about developing huge muscles. You simply want to build the same muscle as a normal, healthy twenty-year-old would have. For specifics on how to plan a weight-training program and how to execute the following exercises properly, see the section entitled "Building Young Muscle" in my last book, *Guide to Turning Back the Clock*.

BENEFIT

Increases metabolism: All muscles have the same metabolism, but if you train and build up a particular muscle, then it will have a faster metabolism. For example, if you're already a cyclist, weight training will increase the metabolism of the leg muscles you use most. According to Cliff Sheats, author of *Lean Bodies,* you can increase metabolism for hours after you exercise. "You will keep your metabolism up for 12 hours after you've strength trained," says Cliff. Cliff recommends strength training and aerobics. He stresses that strength training should be done before aerobics, because "during strength training you're using glycogen as your primary fuel source. After strength training you should do your aerobics because your heart rate will already be up and you've used the glycogen so now you will burn more fatty acid. You'll get to those fat stores better."

MACHINES OR FREE WEIGHTS

If you're not athletic, haven't ever lifted before, or have limited time, start your programs with a good line of weight-training machines in a gym. They're all you ever need for a fast, efficient workout. Cybex and Hammer Strength are two excellent lines to look for when you are shopping for a gym. If you're afraid of injury or intimidated by lifting actual weights, consider a system that works on the hydraulic principle, such as Kaiser. The advantage is that you are simply pressing against hydraulic pressure so that if you falter at any point, the weights won't come crashing down. I have my eighty-three-year-old mother using the Kaiser system three times a week and she loves it! You can progress to the point that a barbell at home will suffice after four to six weeks at the gym.

FAT-BURNING MUSCLES

Since most muscles burn the same number of calories per pound, you could build more of any muscle you choose. But if your choice were a forearm or calf muscles, you would have to spend an inordinate amount of time and painful effort to achieve any result at all. Alternatively, you could choose muscles that are easy to develop quickly, muscles that will grow to a large size. Take the biggest muscle in the upper body, called the latissimus. Pull-ups or lat pull-downs both develop these massive back muscles.

SHOULDER AND BACK

The deltoids and the lats are the only muscles that will give you the accentuated V frame of a lean, muscular individual. Combined with fat loss around your belly, the V frame will dramatically change your shape. In several months you will look much trimmer. In fact, with the extra muscle, you may appear much "thinner" than someone who has lost a great deal more fat. Because that individual has also lost muscle, they're likely to look dumpy, where you can look lean and elegant. Many overweight people are disappointed in how they look after weight loss: tired, haggard, and flabby. Add new muscle and you'll look terrific long before you've lost all the fat you want to.

Deltoids

These muscles drape over the top of your shoulder onto your upper arm to fill out your shoulder and the top of the "V."
  Exercises:
* Overhead presses
* Shoulder shrugs
* Vertical row

Back

This is a huge, largely ignored, area that can provide an enormous opportunity for building fat-burning muscle. When your arm and chest muscles are as large as they'll get, this is fertile new ground to plow. Back muscles assist the abdominal muscles in providing support and stability for your spine.

If you haven't worked on these muscles before, expect big gains. Exercises:
- Chin-ups
- Lat pull-downs

CHEST
The pure bulk in your chest muscles makes them the key fat-burning muscles. They are unique in that so many different exercises can hit them so effectively from so many different directions for terrific development.

Exercises:
- Bench press
- Incline press
- Parallel dips

ARMS
Triceps

These muscles make up the biggest muscle mass in your arm, forming two-thirds of its bulk. If you don't train them, you'll never appear to have decent-sized arms. As muscles with large bulk, they're a great way to build youth and easily outrank the biceps. Women will find this a great way to tighten up any sagging under the back of the upper arm.

Exercises:
- Triceps dips
- Triceps push-down
- Seated triceps press

Biceps

There is a case to be made that rowing exercises for the back and pull-ups develop the biceps sufficiently, so you may not need to do separate biceps exercises if you're pressed for time. Because the biceps recover so quickly, you can use them one day for chin-ups and still be

recovered adequately to use them for rows the next. If you're having trouble with chin-ups, try these exercises first to build up the biceps:
Exercises:
- Standing barbell
- Preacher curl

LEGS

The buttocks, thighs, and calves form the greatest muscle mass in the body and give you the biggest opportunity for building fast-burning muscle.
Exercise:
- Leg Press★★★★

ABDOMINALS

The abdominals are the most powerful stabilizing muscles of the back, and are the most crucial muscles for maintaining that flat washboard abdomen. They're a surprisingly good calorie-burning furnace. You'll do sit-ups and crunches until you're old and gray before you develop that washboard look, so go for the machines.

Abdominal Crunch Machines
- Cybex
- AB Flexor

part five Perfect Weight Control

The Glucose Epidemic

There is a worldwide epidemic of disease spread by an overload of glucose in the diet. It is responsible for sprawling waistlines throughout the United States and Europe and in urban centers from Asia, Africa, and the Middle East to South America. But nowhere has the overload of glucose had a more disastrous consequence than in the Indians of Arizona, where more of the population is overweight than anywhere on earth. But glucose overload hasn't just led to extra pounds; it has caused the most severe epidemic of diabetes ever reported. So common are the amputations in adult diabetics that when asked how diabetes is treated, children answer, "They cut off your limbs." The kidney failure that comes with diabetes is so severe that dialysis centers are filled to overflowing two shifts a day, six days a week. In a single generation, life expectancy has dropped as much as forty years in a single family.

However, Native Americans ate 25 grams of soluble fiber a day for over eight thousand years with remarkable health benefits. Ethnobotanist Gary Nabhan of the Arizona Desert Museum calculated that value by measuring the fiber content of fossilized stool specimens from those millennia. If it seems like a real stretch to eat that amount of fiber, remember that it is our Western diet that is considered dysfunctional . . . a diet that has unleashed a worldwide epidemic of obesity, diabetes, heart disease, and cancer . . . the culinary equivalent of quick sex.

Some of you may object to the concept of food as drugs. Angelo Joaquin Jr., a Tohono O'odham Indian, corrected me when I referred to foods as medicines. He said, "Foods are health." In a very real sense he's right. If you eat a traditional Western diet, you may have many of the attributes of sickness such as high blood sugar, high insulin level, high blood pressure, high cholesterol levels, and low levels of antioxidants. By eating the right foods, all of those signs of illness may disappear. The foods truly can act like medicines. However, for those who always ate the right foods, the foods embodied great good health, not medicinal qualities. So as you make the transition to the right foods, they stop acting as medicines and start delivering health.

Conventional Wisdom
Carbo-load.

LEAN
Spare the carbos.

ROAD MAP
The Indians of Arizona may seem remote and without application to the rest of us. But a close look at these Indians shows how the wrong genes and the wrong foods lead to massive increases in body fat and the tremendous toll the Western diet can take on the most susceptible populations. But more important, even in the face of tremendous genetic adversity, the Pima demonstrate how foods are the most powerful and effective weapons we know to shed body fat and prevent diabetes. The Indians of Arizona are the ultimate acid test for the hypothesis that foods are drugs. Foods that work for them can work wonders for the rest of us even if we're as little as five to ten pounds overweight. This chapter will outline the catastrophe that has befallen the Pima Indians of Arizona and show how the foods that have worked for them can work for you.

THE PIMA
At thirty-five, 90 percent of the Pima are overweight and 50 percent have diabetes. Today they have the highest documented incidence of diabetes on earth, fifteen times higher than the U.S. population as a whole. The type of diabetes they suffer from, Type II, is the leading complication of being overweight.

The Pima Indians became the very first Americans when they

crossed the Bering Strait over thirty thousand years ago. Now you would think that given all the choice North American real estate available at the time, they would have selected beachfront property in Laguna Niguel, California, or something near the slopes in Aspen. Instead they chose the harsh environment of the Arizona desert. But it was a tremendously farsighted or fortuitous strategy that ensured their survival into the late twentieth century, because it was only there that special foods grew which protected them from their genetic destiny. How tough was life in the desert? Summer air temperatures reached 120 degrees. With a surface temperature of 200 degrees, it wasn't too different from being baked in a hot dry oven. Farmers from the great plains scoffed at the idea of growing anything in the desert: Too hot, too dry, alkaline soil, they said. Small wonder. Solar radiation was so fierce, any normal plant was sucked dry. Rainfall rarely reached 3 inches a year. Willing to give it a try? A U.S. Indian agent made these observations of the Pima living in Arizona in the last century: "Place the same number of whites on a barren, sandy desert such as they live on, and tell them to subsist there; the probability is that in two years they would become extinct." On a mountain bike at midday, I was sucked dry within the hour.

Researchers believe that the Pima survived because they had two special genetic traits. First, their intestines and hormones could metabolize the harsh desert foods. According to ethnobotanist Gary Nabhan, the hypothesis is that the Pimas are endowed with a gastrointestinal and endocrine system that may have been selected, in an evolutionary sense, to metabolize the many slow-release complex-carbohydrate foodstuffs available in arid zones. Second, they carried the "thrifty gene," which allowed them to suck nutrients out of a stone when the pickings were slim. It was as if they were bred for the desert. In fact they may have been. Anthropologists believe that before the Pima came to America, they lived in one of the great Asian deserts. This thrifty gene allowed them to survive famine by conserving energy and hoarding stores of fat. When they happened upon the rare feast, usually a wild animal, they couldn't carry it back for storage in the freezer. Instead, they would feast on it in the field. Their genes allowed them to stock away the maximum amount of calories until the next kill. But, when they encountered a kill on a daily basis in the form of burgers at the local drive-through, the thrifty gene grasped for every last calorie when there were far too many calories to be had . . . like a once wretched Dickensian street urchin allowed to feast for years at the king's table. While the human body could adapt to starvation, it couldn't adapt to plenty. This brought the Pima to the ravages of obesity in times of plenty.

In the nineteenth century the Pima were an amazingly fit and highly skilled desert people who built an entire network of irrigation canals on their rivers, the Gila and the Salt. For millennia before, the Pima lived on wild food plants from mesquite pods, tree cholla, prickly pear, cactus, and chia seeds to acorns from live oaks. They farmed amaranth, corn, and their native tepary bean and fished in the Gila. But the end began after the gold rush of 1849. White men tapped water from the Gila, upstream from the Pima land. When their irrigation system ran dry, the Pima were forced to abandon farming. Between 1875 and 1945, the Pima way of life underwent a drastic change. Trading posts appeared on the reservation; sugar and lard became regular commodities, and gradually greens started to disappear from their diet. Wild game was replaced with beef and pork lard. Grease frying was introduced, and the rest, as they say, is history. Not unlike the school lunch programs of the 1950s, the U.S. government began providing them with commodity foods — lard and flour — to relieve their hunger. The government might as well have poisoned them. The tremendous natural genetic advantages for desert survival turned savagely against them. When exposed to high-fat, high-glucose foods, appropriately called "blood mud" or "heart goo," those same genes pried out every last calorie, and held it with a vise-like grip. Some gained over a hundred pounds on U.S. relief goods, ominously foreshadowing, for millions of Americans, the most explosive mixture of foodstuffs imaginable . . . fat and flour — a combination that caused the fastest, biggest weight gain in American and British history during the 1980s, a combination that has made Americans the fattest people of all industrial nations. Fat primed the pump, but the tremendous glucose load from pounds of white flour sealed their fate.

You may be saying to yourself, "How in the world can a population of people who are almost all fat and have beat the world's record for diabetes be great role models for anyone trying to control their weight?" By looking at who the Pima were and who they have become simply through the foods they ate.

When the Pima settled in Arizona, they had the great good fortune of lucking into land that, while incredibly inhospitable to the rest of mankind, was a perfect place for them to thrive. The special Pima foods, found only in the desert, are what protected them against obesity and diabetes. In a remote mountainous area in the Sierra Madre of northwestern Mexico live another population of Pima who are still protected because they eat traditional foods. They are rail thin and hearty. I talked with their chief, Jose Angel Galaviz. At age sixty-four, he works from 6 A.M. to 10 P.M. with so much energy he stops only because it is too dark to work. He is hale and full of good cheer. Farther up the road I talked with a 106-year-old Pima who looked thirty years younger. These Pima weigh an average sixty pounds less than their Arizona cousins. Their diet is extremely simple and incredibly powerful, giving them boundless energy to work their land. The men were involved in activities requiring heavy labor — farming, road construction, wood milling, and fence building. The main sources of protein and carbohydrate are four varieties of beans eaten with corn or flour tortillas. I found I could bike hours through the rugged Sierra Madre on a small meal of beans and tortillas. My appetite was easily killed. I shed extra fat in days and my brain never felt better. Jose uses foods as drugs. He eats more protein in the morning for mental energy, then increases the carbohydrate in the evening as a natural soporific. He rarely eats meat or poultry. A substantial consumption of beans and tortillas gives him a very high level of dietary fiber to cut hunger for extraordinarily long periods. Dr. Mauro Valencia, who visited the Pima along with me, measured their fiber intake at an amazing 100 grams a day.

A National Institutes of Health team led by Dr. Eric Ravussin dissected out of this life in the mountains the most important medicinal property of their diet, an exceptional substance called "slow-release factor" that protected them against obesity and diabetes. Here's how

Dr. Ravussin described it: "The diet has a high concentration of soluble fibers and a type of starch called amylose that is digested very slowly." These fibers form gels and gums in the intestine that have very powerful medicinal effects. You can think of gels and gums as providing a protective layer for your intestine that prevents the swings in blood sugar that make you fat and slow down the digestive process to delay the onset of hunger. Dr. Robert Livingston, the diabetes control officer at the Indian Health Service Hospital, agrees: "These foods act like a medicine by forming a special gel-fiber that slows the sugar release into your blood. They control cholesterol and fat in your bloodstream." Dr. Ravussin and his team hit gold, the magic foods that kept the Mexican Pima thin and healthy, the most vulnerable of all populations to the high-fat, high-sugar, low-fiber Western diet.

Think of this gel as a prophylactic for the intestine. Taken before terrible foods, it blunts their effects by preventing blood sugars from going too high. Here's the proof. Dr. Alberto C. Frati-Munari gave 100 grams of broiled prickly pear leaves before each meal to eight healthy, fourteen obese, and seven diabetic subjects for ten days. Prickly pear, a pearlike fruit that tastes like a strawberry, is a traditional Pima food with a very high soluble-fiber content. Young prickly pear pads are called nopals or *nopalitos*. After the prickly pear intake, he found a significant reduction of cholesterol and triglycerides. Body weight decreased in both the obese and diabetic participants. High blood sugar decreased a mean of 63.4 mg/dl in diabetics and 3.86 mg/dl even in nondiabetics. "For whatever reasons," says Dr. Livingston, "the traditional foods offer protective effects. By modern standards, the traditional diet is ideal. It's not only good in terms of the natural benefits, but it has a great breakdown of fat, carbohydrate, and protein." At one time the Pima Indians may have consumed more legumes per capita per day than any other ethnic population in the world, many loaded with the protective slow-release factor.

Ironically, precisely the same ingredient that protected the Pima from diabetes and obesity also protected the plants themselves from the harsh desert climate. The North American desert floras are rich in edible legumes as well as in cacti and small seeds. These foods are loaded with slow-release factors. Cactus and other desert foods use the gel to hold water when it rains by slowing moisture vapor loss, so they can store the water for use in their fleshy core during the long dry periods. This same gel that allows desert plants to survive punishing months of bone-dry weather forms the viscous protective layer in the intestine of human beings, meting out a small but steady supply of nutrients to the body instead of the sudden and catastrophic rush that fast foods deliver. Just as the plants of the desert had to preserve their water for long periods without rain, so too the Pima preserved each meal and extended its effect over many hours. The consumption of few calories gave them great satiety and long-lived energy. The more the NIH looked, the more foods they found with this protective gel. Mesquite, the Pima's most important wild food, contains a viscous gel called galactomannan in its seeds and pods, which has been shown to lower blood sugar. Opuntia cactus pads, flower buds, and fruit also lower blood sugar. The Pima historically utilized the seeds of a number of plants known to have mucilaginous seed coats, including peppergrass, Indian wheats, chias, and tansy-mustards. The most famous is the legendary tepary bean.

How do you identify foods with slow-release factor? They're not on the package label. But there are two telltale signs of a food with the slow-release factor. First, look for a low glycemic index, or GI, which means that the foods cause a small rise in blood sugar. On a scale of 1 to 100, most Pima foods barely reach 30. Second, look for a high amount of fiber. Soluble fiber has the most powerful slow-releasing effects. For instance, cholla buds have an astounding 21.74 grams of soluble fiber, while saguaro cactus seeds contain an even more amazing 59.53 grams. Since these foods are widely unavailable, I have prepared an extensive list of foods high in soluble fiber, which you will find in the "Hard Fibers" chapter. Beans and breakfast cereals top the list. There is an address for Native Seeds/SEARCH, a company established to help Native Indians return to a more traditional way of eating, in the Appendix if you wish to order Pima foods. Because of the wide interest that diabetics around the country have in the Pima foods, the chapter "Hard Fibers" has a complete list of more widely available high-fiber foods.

So powerful are these foods that there is a movement afoot to convince the Pima and other Native Americans of the Sonoran Desert back onto the foods of their ancestors. Last fall I had dinner with Felipe, a forty-three-year-old award-winning folklorist, who is a Native American. He asked that his last name not be used. As a child growing up on the reservation in Arizona, he loved seeing the elders in his village. Today, he's distressed that the youngsters have been tragically deprived of the opportunity to learn from the old members of their tribe. "Our grandparents," Felipe says, "were great historians and great story-tellers. Our grandparents would tell us about their grandparents. My grandparents' generation lived to be over a hundred years old, but my parents' generation is dying before our eyes, as is even our own. When I was growing up in the 1960s I always saw the elders. Today I do not see any of them. They have been erased from the villages. My grandparents and great-grandparents had their own garden; my parents did not. My grandmother told me stories about how she would go to her grandmother's house and care for her garden. She would irrigate her watermelon, corn, beans, and squash. It is my parents' generation that stopped eating the traditional foods."

Felipe now spends his days educating his people about the traditional desert foods and how they can use these foods to prevent and control obesity and diabetes. The genius of the Native Seeds/ SEARCH Project is how they market the traditional diet. "We're not just reinforcing a good diet, but a value of their culture," says Kevin Dahl, education director at Native Seeds/SEARCH. Throughout the American Sonoran Desert, you will find cluster upon cluster of Felipe's converts. It is only through their coalescence that the great peoples of the desert can survive. It may be only through Felipe's message that the rest of us will stem the tide of coronary artery disease, obesity, cancer, and diabetes that is washing across America. To this day, the Pima still receive U.S. relief goods that are little improvement over the flour and lard of yesteryear. Those include canned meat with a large layer of fat packed on top, processed cheese, white flour, canned milk, and peanut butter. This food is distributed free of charge. The government might as well have planted land mines, judging by the terrible amputations you see throughout the native villages. Although Western foods had a pronounced and catastrophic effect on the desert Indians, their effect on the American public may not be as uniformly visible, but it is just as tragic and nearly as widespread. Food is the number-one cause of death in America. What ruined the Pima can kill you, but foods that allowed the Pima to live into their hundreds can perfectly control your weight, greatly improve your health, and extend your longevity.

Will the Pima foods work for you? In Australia, Caucasians were put on a Pima diet, and researchers found a dramatic drop in blood sugar and cholesterol levels, and even a boost in immune system function. In this study eight healthy Australian Caucasian men and women (aged twenty-one to twenty-four) were fed six traditional River Pima staple foods: lima beans, white tepary beans, yellow tepary beans, mesquite pods, corn, and acorns. The Pima Indian foods caused little increase in blood sugar or insulin response, whereas Western staples such as potatoes, bread, and other processed cereal products generated high blood sugars and insulin responses. This is the first study to confirm that the particular legumes (lima beans, tepary beans, and mesquite pods) that dominated the Pima Indian diet are also slow-release. This further supports the theory that the traditional foods were an important factor in protecting indigenous populations from developing diabetes and obesity. All six meals were digested significantly more slowly than was the Western counterpart, white bread. Acorns, which were particularly high in fiber, had the lowest digestibility. The glycemic indices of these foods were all low, ranging from 16 for acorns to 40 for corn compared to 100 for white bread. The slow-release factor protected both Pima and Caucasians.

HARD BODIES

In Arizona to this day there are still hunter-gatherers, but they are white men. They are rail thin, with the gaunt tough faces of the cowboys of yesteryear. They pitch tents in the desert, hunt rabbit, deer, and pig. They live off the golden foods of the desert, from mesquite soup to prickly pear. You will see them on the street corners in Tucson selling the *Arizona Daily Star* in the mornings. They retire to their tents in the desert during the afternoon. These men live close to the ground. They live a hard life, foraging for food and struggling for money, but their gaunt figures belie the secrets of the Arizona desert. They have hard bodies because they gather and eat hard foods the hard way.

21

True Confessions

OK. So you think: "What does this guy know about dieting. He's 6 percent body fat and probably never had an extra ounce of body fat on him in his life." Wrong! Like most people who are lean, I have had to work at it remarkably hard. In fact, one reason for writing *Perfect Weight Control* was to figure out how to deal with the constant worry about maintaining weight while following a crazy schedule, for my family, my colleagues, and myself. As proof of my concept, I deliberately gained 18.5 pounds for this book . . . not muscle, but fat . . . from 190 pounds to 208.5 pounds. Fat! How did I do it? By breaking every rule in the book. To really punch up my weight quickly, I looked for any high-glucose carbos and high-fat foods. I could put on five pounds overnight if I wished . . . ice cream, jelly donuts, cream cheese and bagels. But what alarmed me was that when I got serious about losing the weight, my weight continued to soar. I stuck hard by the low-fat food approach — only to discover that those low-fat foods were of the moderate- and high-glucose variety.

But once I wrestled my weight problem to the floor by dumping my glucose load, my motivation soared. I could lose half a pound a day any day I wanted, week in, week out. Not only did I avoid the lethargy and dopiness of dieting, but my energy and motivation soared. In the end I found a remarkably simple application of the principles in this book. I chose the Sonoran diet described in the "Hard Cuisine" chapter. Here's what worked and why.

For breakfast, I had a protein shake, usually Met Rx, to kill my hunger. That obliterated my hunger through a long morning bike ride up until well after noon. On days I couldn't exercise in the morning, I had a glass of skim milk followed by a bowl of high-fiber cereal, usually Fiber One or an undercooked oatmeal. At lunch, I'd eat a whole wheat burrito with wild rice and black beans followed by three side orders of black beans. True, it took me several weeks to work my way up to all those beans without side effects, but once I made it, I was truly astounded. The bean and rice meal, basic nutrition to four billion people around the world, obliterated my hunger through the afternoon and evening and gave me the mental energy and physical stamina to make it to midnight. Even then I'd have to hit myself with a sledgehammer to go to sleep. In the late afternoon I might have an all-oat granola bar, but that was it until bedtime. Then I'd have a single piece of chocolate. That's it. I weighed myself every morning on waking and every evening before going to bed. I found it strong motivation to keep myself going. To see that scale showing half a pound less every morning that I followed this schedule was like watching a small miracle . . . perfect weight control without the pain. On evenings that I had to have a business dinner, I'd order a single piece of fish. The high-fiber load left over from lunch gave me great control throughout dinner. The fish was super-filling and kept me alert well into the evening. I did add some cantaloupe in the morning and some veggies with lunch once my pattern was established. My diet was so successful that I kept going past my original target, 190 pounds, toward my high school weight of 184. I'd caution you that this was part of a solid workout program, so I wasn't starving myself or doing myself any harm by overshooting. On airplanes, I took a bag of oats and a big container of plain, low-fat yogurt. The combination was filling enough to all but eliminate airline cuisine on a fairly hefty travel schedule.

For my exercise program, I simply punched up the intensity . . . no more time or distance, just pumping up my heart rate five or six times in long intervals up some hills. I easily shed twelve pounds in the first three weeks of increased intensity . . . virtually all of it fat. If my energy fell, I'd boost my low-glucose carbos by 200 calories a day. That's all it took, and my brain could really feel the difference since it becomes so sensitive to the druglike effects of carbos.

My favorite newfound foods were beans, a remarkable and singular tool to control your appetite anytime, anywhere. I swear that after three helpings of beans, I'm just not hungry for a good twelve hours. I may crave a little chocolate, but that's easily purged with just a square or two, sucked gently because my stomach is so full. In fact, if I was to summarize my success into a catchy title for a fad weight-loss book, I'd call it Dr. Bob's Bike and Bean Diet, because bikes and beans are the best two ingredients I've come across yet to control your weight perfectly.

Protein is the other superweapon that kills hunger and energizes me. I found that really drastically cutting all the medium- and fast-burning carbos, my weight dropped like a stone. Like many fit Americans, I was plagued by ring-around-the-belly fat that just wouldn't go away no matter how intense my training. Dropping my glucose load did the trick. I did momentarily fall into the trap of eating a lot more fat to cut down my glucose load, but that backfired and I just got fat again.

I also picked the right time of year. By working in the spring on changes in your food intake to foods that make you thin and gradually increasing your fitness, you're ready to strip off the fat come July 1. Use this month to drop your weight. If you find yourself really hankering for carbos, reread the chapter "Make Your Brain Feel Great" to take every available measure to get your serotonin up so you don't need to use food to keep it there.

Even with a major setback, recovery was easy because I didn't crave foods and my physiology remained that of fat loss. I fell into the typical trap on a trip home from overseas and found my weight pop up by two pounds from airline food, but after three days back on the program, I was back where I belonged.

Now I feel like a teenager again. Stripping off all the extra weight lets me spring to the net in tennis, pounce to the top of the hill in front of the pack on a bike . . . and fit into suits I haven't worn since college. The best part about it is knowing that I have a secret weapon that I can pull out anytime, anywhere, and that bringing my weight back under control will be a pleasure not a burden.

22

Postscript

We stand on the cusp of a spectacular new era of weight control that is intellectually fascinating and scientifically dazzling. Weight control has become a thinking man's and thinking woman's game. This book has all the basic tools to enter the dawn of this new era. That begins with using foods as the drugs that can make you look and feel the way you've always wanted. By making your brain feel great, you grasp the willpower to eat the foods that make you lean. By killing your hunger, you grasp the ultimate self-control over bingeing and overeating. By controlling your glucose load, you shut down the hormones that make you fat. The arsenal of powerful foods presented is the rich and plentiful pharmacy of the future. Feedforward Eating puts it all together into a timetable for eating so that you feel great and perform your best all day long. Hard cuisines let you put the principles of perfect weight control to work in terrific meals from the world's healthiest and leanest cultures. By following these fundamentals, you'll notice a marked drop in body fat and a turn to a far healthier way of eating and living.

When I read sections of this book to my father, he took me aside. As a Harvard-trained psychiatrist and a practitioner for fifty years, he said, "Do me one favor, don't give people an impossible goal, don't tell them a weight they have to reach. It only creates misery." For that reason you won't find recommended weights. If you follow all the advice given in this book you will settle in on a very comfortable livable weight that is in perfect balance with your body's metabolism and at which you will feel terrific. Chances are, you'll be trimmer than if you settled on a number taken from a table of recommended weights.

As your body fat drops, you will achieve a wonderful feeling of self-control, and a sense of command. You'll finally feel fully in charge of your physical life. You will feel strikingly different than you do under traditional diets: calm and energetic, without the hunger or anxiety that comes with food deprivation. You are now empowered — through the most advanced and effective foods ever known to control your weight in a healthy and enjoyable way — to become the best you've ever been: trimmer, fitter, smarter, better motivated, with a winning attitude and a terrific mood from dawn to dusk. You don't have to wait for the latest genetically engineered drugs. If foods can keep the Pima thin, the people with the most severe genetic predisposition to obesity on earth, they can work a small miracle for you. Look at this as a terrific adventure across the span of time, geography, distant cultures, and powerful spiritual beliefs. I'd wish you good luck, but you won't need it, for the foods in this book contain the motivation, staying power, and druglike qualities to make you look and feel great. Embark on these changes with confidence, high hopes, and a great spirit.

For each of the chapters listed below, you'll find additional information, resources, and more complete descriptions of items discussed in the book.

Chapter 4: Make Your Brain Feel Great
Food supplement

PMS Escape is manufactured by InterNutria of Lexington, Massachusetts. If you can't find it in your health food store, you can call 800-PMS-6369 to order it over the phone. A one-month supply comes in a box of eight packets and costs $12.95.

SPECIAL NOTE: Since the therapy is limited to just several days in each menstrual cycle, women are not likely to gain too much weight with PMS. The advantage is that by drinking pure carbos, severe PMS sufferers avoid bingeing on the fat-laden carbos that cause an even greater weight gain.

Devices

DayLIGHT bright light   This is a flicker-free 120 watt diffused light source with three brightness settings — 10,000 lux, 7,500 lux, and 3,500 lux ($425).

PillowLIGHT dawn simulator   This device will simulate natural dawn ($375; controller, $425).

QuadrixLIGHT   This combines the DayLIGHT and PillowLIGHT ($2,495). SphereOne says, "This emulates the quality and changing light of a natural day. This artificial window begins the day by slowly bringing the lowest sitting horizon module to full brightness. And then, while maintaining a high illumination level throughout, the primary light slowly progresses to overhead modules following the natural movement of the sun from horizon to azimuth and returning back to the horizon module at the end of the day. You are literally working under the clock of an artificial sky."

The above items are manufactured by SphereOne.

To get information on SphereOne's products you can write or call them at:

SphereOne, Inc.
20 Easedale Road
Wayne, NJ 07470
201-942-9772

FreshAIR negative ionizer   This comes in a portable model, worn as a pendant or in your shirt pocket ($150) or as a desktop model ($120), to be placed on your desk. Ion output is 1.6 trillion ions/se/cm at 2.5 cm.

Chapter 6:   Drop Your Glucose Load
How to Lower Insulin Levels

The most elusive holy grail of diet researchers has been a way to increase the burning of fat. By decreasing insulin levels, researchers at Duke University can light up and switch on the receptors on fat cells to do just that. A rock-steady low-insulin level is the single most important goal for maintaining an ideal weight. Decreasing your glucose load is the biggest step; however, these additional measures will get your insulin down and keep it down to speed fat loss.

Frequent small meals   Smaller, more frequent meals have an enormous impact on insulin levels. Fasting morning insulin levels drop 25 to 30 percent, allowing you to begin losing weight without dieting by unlocking fat stores. A number of experts recommend eating five smaller than usual meals throughout the day rather than the standard three meals per day. The most prominent is Professor David Jenkins. His classic study, entitled *Nibbling Versus Gorging,* found that cholesterol was lowered by increasing meal frequency alone, with no alteration in the nature or the amount of food eaten. However, by increasing the intake of soluble fiber and eating low glycemic index carbos, you achieve a quite dramatic lowering of insulin levels and weight loss.

More frequent meal advocates only add a couple of more meals to the traditional fare, but what happens if you really go crazy with the nibbling routine? Men who eliminated traditional meals and instead ate seventeen snacks per day over the course of two weeks decreased their serum insulin level by 27.9 percent and the key stress hormone, cortisol, by 17.3 percent, compared to men eating three squares. The decrease in cortisol may reflect the much lower stress that nibbling takes on your body.

Beware that when these grazing studies first hit the popular media, they created a weight gain free-for-all. What better combination, figured the unwitting reader, than daylong grazing on low-fat foods. The trouble is that these low-fat foods were the super-fast-burning carbohydrates that pump up insulin levels and hunger levels to prompt the massive overconsumption that has so fattened America. Many Americans mistook grazing for high-powered mowing through any foods that come across their path. These snacks must be properly constructed minimeals that include protein and slow-burning carbos. Here's an example: A garden burger, constructed from fresh mushrooms, onion, rolled oats, brown rice, bulgur wheat, low-fat mozzarella cheese, and nonfat cottage cheese on a seven grain bread. I like the taste better than a beef burger. Its quieting effect on the metabolism makes it a double pleasure.★★★★★

Wine   Very dry wines may lower your insulin level. I'm not a big fan of this technique, but if you are a real wine aficionado and must have your wine, go for the very dry ones that are helping the cause. Be wary of hard liquor, which increases insulin levels.★★★

Aerobic exercise   A single bout of exercise can reduce your insulin level. UCLA researchers demonstrated that forty-five minutes of exercise had the same effect on lowering blood sugar as a single maximum injection of insulin. Exercise does that by using each contraction to suck sugar into the muscle without the need to make more insulin. The adrenaline rush of exercise also suppresses the release of insulin. Even after you've toweled off and showered, insulin continues to work more effectively, so you need less of it for an additional twenty-four hours. Over the long term, insulin increases the number of insulin receptors, so the insulin you make is more effective and you can get away with lower levels of it.

Weight training   An increased muscle mass provides a bigger dumping ground for blood sugar so that you can dump more of it there instead of into fat stores. Look at the muscle as a huge protective buffer against rising blood sugar levels. There's a whole chapter on weight training, called "Building a Fat-Burning Engine."★★★★

Mental firepower   The hormone adrenaline stimulates fat breakdown in the area that counts most, the fat in your abdomen. Researchers discovered that the more adrenaline you produce in a twenty-four-hour period, the less intra-abdominal fat you have. Who has a higher adrenaline level? Those who get higher levels of mental stimulation during the day through a busy, confident, active lifestyle. These same people have lower insulin levels.★★★★★

Less aspartame   Foods alone don't make insulin rise; the anticipation of incoming calories can also cause a rise in insulin. Jim Heffley, Ph.D., who heads the Nutrition Counseling Service in Austin, Texas, says, "I think what the aspartame is doing is that there is a rise in insulin level as a response to the sweet taste. Soon after, the insulin goes down because there's nothing there for it to work on. That initial insulin response makes you hungry."★★★★

Change medications   The following medications are also known to raise insulin levels. If you have a high insulin level, ask your doctor if there are other medications that would work just as well.

- Thiazide diuretics: Known colloquially as water pills, these are very commonly used to treat high blood pressure.
- Beta blockers: Although there are dozens of uses for beta blockers, they are most commonly used to treat high blood pressure, certain irregular heart rhythms, and as prevention for a recurrent heart attack.

Supplements That Lower Insulin Levels   Supplements are widely touted as a valid way to decrease insulin levels. The scientific validity of some claims is on pretty shaky ground. However, some supplements do make the insulin in your system more effective. If you only take supplements to increase insulin efficiency and continue eating high-glucose carbohydrates, you would expect them to make you fatter, because you're using all of your excess insulin at its maximum advantage to store fat. However, if you follow many of the above recommendations to decrease insulin levels, then these supplements may coax your body into making even less insulin. These supplements are not a mainstay, but may give a modest boost to your efforts. Fish oils, vanadyl sulphate, chromium, and magnesium are the key insulin-lowering supplements. C. Roland Kahn, M.D., research director of the Joslin Diabetes Center in Boston, warns, "Regarding this class of agents, it's important to note that there is a lot of anecdotal information, but they should be regarded as experimental and should only be taken with a physician's approval because they can all be toxic in high doses."

Fish oil: The Garvin Institute in Australia demonstrated that the Omega 3 fatty acids, which are found in fish oils, allow your body to do with less insulin. Your body can also manufacture these fatty acids from a supplement called flax oil. Flax oil allows your muscles to build a membrane where insulin can move sugar into cells far more effectively. Fish, however, are a far more effective source of Omega 3 fatty acids. In one highly amusing experiment, food technologists fed fish oils to pigs so that the quality of their bacon would be higher. That is, the bacon would have a higher amount of good fats. It worked, but the bacon smelled so much like fish that it was deemed inedible.★★

Chromium: This was last year's hottest supplement, promoted for its ability to "burn fat." It does no such thing. However, it can help you lower your insulin levels, and for that it is a very worthwhile supplement. Chromium expert Richard Anderson of the USDA's Agricultural Research Service recently presented the results of a study that showed that people in China with Type II diabetes had marked reductions in their blood sugar and insulin levels after two to four months of taking chromium picolinate supplements.

The volunteers in his study, who received a total of 1000 mcg daily, improved their glucose levels significantly after only two months, compared to the placebo group. The low-chromium group — those volunteers getting a total of 200 mcg daily — showed no significant difference in blood glucose from the placebo group.

Both the 1000 mcg and the 200 mcg chromium groups had a significant drop in plasma insulin just two months after beginning the supplements, and a further drop at four months. People with Type II, or maturity-onset, diabetes produce more insulin than normal in the early stages of the disease, Anderson explained, because the hormone is less efficient at clearing glucose from the blood. Chromium apparently makes the hormone more efficient.

Beware that chromium may not be a free ride. The scientific publication of the Federation of American Societies of Experimental Biology reported damage to chromosomes of human cells grown in tissue cultures. Critics assert that researchers used up to 6,200 times more chromium picolinate than found in a supplement. But because a single dose remains in a mouse cell for sixty-four days, there is the risk of accumulating toxic amounts with daily supplements. The National Academy of Sciences maintains that 50 to 200 micrograms daily is a "safe and adequate intake."

Also, if you're already overweight, the chromium helps your body store blood sugar more efficiently, it makes insulin work better, and it could make you fatter if you take lots of it. Sound crazy? Dr. John Ivy of the University of Texas at Austin ran a study in which dieting women took 400 milligrams of chromium a day. They gained so much weight, they dropped out of the study. Combined with the wrong foods, it's a disaster. But as part of a terrific diet, it can lower insulin and glucose levels to help you lose weight. Taking chromium with a high refined sugar diet is a little like an alcoholic on two gallons of Ripple secretly believing that a glass of red wine is going to make him healthier!

Vanadyl sulphate: This substance is a rare metal that is present in the earth's crust. Most people get a little bit of it from their diet because it is present in anything that's got earth salts in it — like meat and vegetables. In the supplement form, you receive about 1,000 times more than you would ever get in a diet. C. Ronald Kahn, M.D., research director of the Joslin Diabetes Center in Boston, says, "Vanadyl sulphate improves insulin sensitivity but its mechanism is not known." Two independent trials showed improved insulin sensitivity and in some cases lowering of insulin requirements in Type II, non-insulin-dependent diabetics. In humans, there is no evidence of effect on Type I diabetics. In order for vanadyl sulphate to be effective, you need 125 mg. a day. ★★★

Magnesium: Both the famous Harvard Nurses study and several small clinical trials have shown that magnesium decreases insulin resistance and therefore your insulin level.

Dr. Kahn says, "Magnesium has no beneficial effects specifically related to diabetes. The flaw with making that assumption based on the Harvard Nurses study is that it is an epidemiologic survey where they are trying to correlate the amount of magnesium in the diet with some outcome. They are not talking about supplements.

It's a very indirect measurement. The point is that it's not clear that the effects are due to magnesium."

Drugs That Lower Insulin

Alpha-glucosidase inhibitors: Precose, the only FDA-approved alpha-glucosidase inhibitor, works by slowing the digestion of carbohydrates so that the absorption of sugar is much more gradual. Precose blocks carbo absorption in the upper intestine, but allows it in the lower intestine. This results in a more even and slow absorption of glucose. The real value is in mild diabetes. Precose will not work alone to help you lose weight. If you undertake the full-court dietary press outlined above, Precose will help to lower your insulin level further. Since many diabetic patients are on high-carbohydrate diets, they suffer a very large surge in blood sugars right after each meal. Many existing therapies, insulin included, don't address this problem. Patients treated with precose have blood glucose levels and insulin levels significantly lower than patients treated with a placebo. Chemically, the drug looks like a carbohydrate, so it tricks digestive enzymes in the gut to choose it over carbohydrate with the result that fewer carbohydrates are digested. The drug may have a strong weight-loss function, but only when taken in doses that are unacceptably high for humans. However, the insulin-lowering effect is an important one when added to other measures that lower insulin levels. Dr. David Jenkins emphasizes that the snacking strategy has a similar effect on slowing the absorption rate. Precose only works when taken with food. If you give it to someone who's fasting, it has absolutely no effect.★★★

Antineuropeptide Y: Neuropeptide Y is the brain's single most powerful hormone to increase insulin production and increase hunger for carbohydrates. Some obese people may have a defective switch in the brain that prevents the production of neuropeptide Y from being shut down. This is the nightmare, meltdown scenario for runaway obesity. It could be the major genetic reason that people are fat. The hormone leptin shuts off neuropeptide Y in normal people. In the obese, regardless of how much leptin they make, the leptin doesn't shut down the production of neuropeptide Y. That makes people ravenously hungry and induces a condition called hyperphagia, which, translated, means massive overeating. Millennium Pharmaceuticals, Inc. of Cambridge, Massachusetts, is developing a blocking drug against neuropeptide Y.

Leptin: The brain makes a chemical called neuropeptide Y, which gives you a voracious appetite and increases the production of insulin to make you very fat. The antidote is the hormone leptin, which targets neuropeptide Y, according to Thomas W. Stephens of the Eli Lily Research Laboratories in Indianapolis. Leptin should cut appetite and, more important, cut the amount of insulin that you produce. Leptin has been touted as the most effective potential weight-loss drug ever. It is eagerly awaited by millions. Weight Watchers International says, "If you look at the research, the product allowed the mice to eat less and exercise more effectively — which is exactly what we teach people how to do. The drug could improve business for Weight Watchers." Researchers are beginning clinical trials with leptin, but it is not commercially available.

Ciglitazone and Troglitazone: Both improve insulin sensitivity in muscle and fat so the body does not have to make as much insulin. Diabetes experts predict these will be very important drugs.

Body Fat Insulin Test

Abhimanyu Garg, M.D., an associate professor of internal medicine at the University of Texas Southwestern Medical Center in Dallas, says the best way to "pinch" is to take (with your thumb and forefinger) the skin about an inch to the right or left of the belly button and literally pinch the excess skin between the two fingers. Dr. Garg says, "Do not include the belly button. Make a fold above the muscles — do not include the muscles." If you have 3 cm or 1¼ inches of fat, you are "overfat" and need to lose it.

Chapter 10:   Hard Beans
Boca Burgers

The Boca Burger Company, based in Fort Lauderdale, has products in supermarkets across the country. They have three burgers, all soy based: a vegan original that is no-fat; Chef Max's Favorite, which is 98 percent fat-free; and a Hint of Fresh Garlic, which is 99 percent fat-free. "We give people the fast-food hamburger experience without all the negatives," says owner Max Shonder. To find where Boca Burgers are sold near you, contact

Boca Burger Company
1660 NE 12th Terrace
Fort Lauderdale, FL 33305
954-524-1977

Chapter 13:   Hard Veggies
Devices

The Vita-Mixer Corporation
800-VITAMIX

Chapter 17:   Hard Cuisine

Opposite are comparisons of life expectancy, disease rates, and food intake for the Mediterranean (Greece), America, and Asia (Japan) for the years 1960 and 1991. The year 1960 in Greece is considered the gold standard for dietary outcomes for cancer and heart disease.

Chapter 19:   Fat-Ripping Exercises

Polar Electro Inc.
99 Seaview Boulevard
Port Washington, NY 11050
800-227-1314 or 516-484-2400

	Greece		United States		Japan	
	1960	1991	1960	1991	1960	1991
Life expectancy at 45 years of age*						
MEN	31	32.5	27	31	27	33.3
WOMEN	34	36.7	33	36.3	32	39.1
Coronary heart disease						
MEN	33	133	189	231	34	48.5
WOMEN	14	55.7	54	124	21	27.5
Cerebrovascular disease						
MEN	26	129.3	30	52	102	100.9
WOMEN	23	133.9	24	45.3	57	72.4
Breast cancer						
WOMEN	8	20.6	22	31.6	4	9
Stomach cancer						
MEN	10	13.8	6	7.9	48	51.5
WOMEN	6	7.1	3	3.5	26	22
Colorectal cancer						
MEN	3	11.8	11	22.6	5	23.1
WOMEN	3	12.5	10	22	5	18.9
Total cancers						
MEN	83	219	102	250.6	98	228.1
WOMEN	61	110.5	87	163.4	77	112.8

	Greece		United States		Japan	
	1960	1991	1960	1991	1960	1991
Kilograms per Capita Consumption**						
All Fats	37.4	59.06	43.19	56.13	8.47	27.18
Mainly saturated fat containing oils	0.06	0.01	0.88	0.73	0.26	0.47
Animal fat (including fish oil and butter)	2.22	3.78	11.13	5.68	1.28	2.71
Fruits and fruit products (excluding wine)	160.44	212.22	92.48	148.3	36.4	57.92
Vegetables and vegetable products	89.64	226.94	87.6	116.0	88.05	111.3
Legumes and products	7.87	5.83	3.77	3.45	3.91	2.46
Cereals and products (excluding beer)	167.39	148.74	90.3	113.7	175.13	146.14
Potatoes	31.76	82.41	49.61	58.02	54	28.34
Meat	20.9	72.08	91.6	115.4	7.53	37.98
Fish and seafood and products	19.11	18.4	14.08	21.68	49.31	72.26
Eggs and products	5.75	11.05	18.26	13.69	9.05	18.71
Alcohol	40.24	65.83	68.78	113.9	29.8	75.15

*1992, 1993, 1994 World Health Statistics Annual, WHO, Geneva
**Compiled by Elizabeth Lenart, Ph.D., HSPH. Data provided by the WHO Food and Health Indicators of Europe, 1993. Please note that these foods are consumption-trend data. They reflect what disappears from the marketplace.

Chapter 20: The Glucose Epidemic
Native Seeds/SEARCH
2509 North Campbell Avenue, #325
Tucson, AZ 85719
602-327-9123

Fiber: Fiber is found only in plant foods. There are two types of dietary fiber: soluble fiber dissolves in water and insoluble fiber does not. The fibers called gums, mucilages, and pectin are all soluble. Examples include beans, oats, and apples. Cellulose, hemicellulose, and lignin are insoluble fibers. Examples include whole grains, potatoes, and wheat bran.

Galanin: A protein that influences eating by increasing the body's preference for fats and carbohydrates. Simply put, as galanin increases, so does your desire to eat fatty and high-carbohydrate foods.

Glucagon: A hormone secreted in the pancreas, glucagon is insulin's opposite. While glucagon makes sure the blood sugar levels don't get too low, insulin makes sure that blood sugar levels don't go too high. Glucagon also shifts metabolism into burning mode, while insulin shifts it into storing mode.

Glucose: Glucose is the body's chief source of energy. It is a simple sugar that passes easily into the bloodstream from the digestive tract when we eat carbohydrates. Virtually all carbohydrates can ultimately be broken down into glucose, their lowest common denominator. The term "blood sugar" is actually slang for blood glucose, which is the concentration of glucose in the blood.

Total glucose load: The total sum of all the glucose released from foods that are either made of sugar or convert to sugar in the body. The higher your load, the wilder your blood sugar levels go.

Glycemic index (GI): This index rates carbohydrates for their effect on blood sugar in the body. Rapidly digested foods have a high GI. Slowly digested foods, more desirable for weight loss and health, have a low GI. The greater number or higher GI foods you eat, the higher your total glucose load. For the purposes of clarity, the term glucose load is substituted in this book.

Insulin: A hormone made by the pancreas, insulin helps the body's tissues absorb and use glucose and fats. Insulin plays a role in food cravings by influencing the production of the brain chemical galanin.

Leptin: A hormone produced by fat, leptin plays an important role in how the body manages its fat supply. The amount of leptin in the body correlates to how much fat is stored in the body. Greater levels of leptin are found in individuals with more fat.

MCH (melanin concentrating hormone): This is an appetite stimulating hormone, which is produced in the brain.

Chapter One: Introduction

Barnard, J. Role of diet and exercise in the management of hyperinsulinemia and associated atherosclerotic risk factor. *American Journal of Cardiology,* 69 (1992):440–444.

Chen, J., T.C. Campbell, J. Li, R. Peto. *Diet, Life-style and Mortality in China. A Study of the Characteristics of 65 Chinese Counties.* Oxford: Oxford University Press; Ithaca: Cornell University Press; Beijing: People's Medical Publishing House, 1991.

Concar, David. Bodies: Shape and destiny: What makes some people fat and others thin? *New Scientist* 146 (1974):23–27.

Goldberg, Israel (ed.). *Functional Foods.* New York: Chapman & Hall, 1994.

Kuczmarski, R., et al. Increasing prevalence of overweight among U.S. adults. *JAMA* 272 (1994):205–211.

O'Brien, Lynne T., et al. Effects of a high-complex-carbohydrate low-cholesterol diet plus bran supplement on serum lipids. *Journal of Applied Nutrition,* vol. 37, no. 1 (1985).

Rosen, J.C., et al. Cognitive behavior therapy for negative body image in obese women. *Behavior Therapy* 26 (1995):25–42.

Chapter 3: Foods As Drugs

Blundell, J., V. Burley, and J. Cotton. Dietary fat and the control of energy intake: Evaluating the effects on meal size and post-meal satiety. *American Journal of Clinical Nutrition* 57 (1983):7725–7785.

Blundell, J., and A. Hill. Serotoninergic modulation of the pattern of eating and the profile and hunger-satiety in humans. *International Journal of Obesity* 11 (1987):141–153.

Brewerton, T., M. Heffernan, and N. Rosenthal. Psychiatric aspects of the relationship between eating and mood. *Nutritional Review* 44 (Suppl. May 1986):78–88.

Cabellero, B. Brain serotonin and carbohydrate craving in obesity. *International Journal of Obesity* 11 (1987):179–183.

Christensen, L., and C. Redig. Effect of meal composition on mood. *Behavioral Neurology* 107(2) (1993):246–353.

Cowen, P., I. Anderson, and C. Fairburn. Neurochemical effects of dieting: Relevance to changes in eating and affective disorders. In H. Anderson and S. Kennedy, eds. *Biology of Feast and Famine* 10 (1993):L 269–284.

Delgado, P., et al. Neuroendocrine and behavioral effects of dietary tryptophan restriction in healthy subjects. *Life Sciences* 45 (1989).

Fernstrom, J. Dietary amino acids and brain function. *Journal of American Diet* 94 (1994):71–77.

Leibowitz, S. Neurochemical control of macronutrient intake. In Y. Domura, S. Tarui, S. Donoue, et al., eds. *Progress in Obesity Research.* London: John Libbey, 1991, pp. 13–18.

Shintani, T., et al. The Wai'anae Diet Program: A culturally sensitive, community-based obesity and clinical intervention program for the Native Hawaiian population. *Hawaii Medical Journal* 53(5) (1994):136–141.

Chapter 4: Make Your Brain Feel Great

Banderet, L.E., and H.R. Lieberman. Treatment with tyrosine, a neurotransmitter precursor, reduces environmental stress in humans. *Brain Research Bulletin* 22 (1989):759–762.

Blum, K., P. Sheridan, R.C. Wood, E.R. Braverman, T.J.H. Chen, and D. Comings. Dopamine D2 receptor gene variants: association and linkage studies in impulsive-addictive compulsive behavior. *Pharmacogenetics* 5 (1995):121–141.

Blum, K., E.R. Braverman, and D.E. Comings. Reward Deficiency Syndrome. *American Scientist* 84 (1996):133–145.

Compton, P.A., M.D. Anglin, E. Khalsa, Denison and A. Paredes. The D2 dopamine receptor gene, addiction and personality: Clinical correlates in cocaine abusers. *Biological Psychology* 39 (1966): 302–304, 1996.

Czeisler C.A., A.J. Chiasera, and J.F. Duffy. Research on sleep, circadian rhythms and aging: Applications to manned spaceflight. *Experiments in Gerontology* 26 (1991):217–232.

Epstein, R., et al. Dopamine D4 receptor exon III polymorphism associated with the human personality trait of novelty seeking. *Nature Genetics* 12 (1996):78–80.

Lieberman, H.R., L.E. Banderet, and B. Shukitt-Hale. Tyrosine protects humans from the adverse effects of acute exposure to hypoxia and cold. *Society of Neuroscience Abstracts* 16 (1990):272.

McTavish, D., and R. Heel. Dexfenfluramine: A review of its pharmacological properties and therapeutic potential in obesity. *Drug Evaluation* 43 (1992):713–733.

Noble, E.P. The gene that rewards alcoholism. *Scientific America* 3(2) (1996):52:61.

Principles and Practice of Sleep Medicine. Philadelphia: W.B. Saunders Company, 1993. *See* chapter 95 by Michael Terman.

Rosenthal, N.E. *Winter Blues.* New York: Guilford Press, 1993.

Terman, Michael, and Juan Terman. Treatment of seasonal affective disorder with a high-output negative ionizer. *Journal of Alternative and Complementary Medicine.* Vol. 1, no. 1 (1995).

Williams, R. Neurobiology, cellular and molecular biology, and pyschosomatic medicine. *Psychosomatic Medicine* 56 (1994):308–315.

Wurtman, J. Depression and weight gain: The serotonin connection. *Journal of Affective Disorders* 29 (1993):183–192.

Wurtman, J. The involvement of brain serotonin in excessive carbohydrate snacking by obese carbohydrate cravers. *Journal of American Dietary Association* 84(9) (1984):1004–1007.

Wurtman, J., A. Brezezinski, R. Wurtman, and B. Laferrere. Effect of nutrient intake on premenstrual depression. *American Journal of Obstetrics and Gynecology* 161 (1989):1228–1234.

Chapter 5: Turn Off Hunger

Bray, G., B. York, and J. Delaney. A survey of the opinions of obesity experts on the causes and treatment of obesity. *American Journal of Clinical Nutrition* 55 (1992):151–154S.

Cabanac, M. The physiological role of pleasure. *Science* 173 (1971):1103–1107.

deGraffin, C., T. Hulshof, J.A. Westrate, and P. Jas. Short-term effects of different amounts or protein, fat and carbohydrates on satiety. *American Journal of Clinical Nutrition* 55(1992):33–38.

Gordon, C., and D.S. Grimes. Satiety value of wholemeal and white bread. *Lancet,* July 8, 1978, editorial.

Holt, S.H.A., P. Petocz, E. Farmakalidis, et al. A satiety index of common foods. *European Journal of Clinical Nutrition* 49 (1995): 675–690.

Jenkins, D.J.A., et al. Nibbling versus gorging: Metabolic advantages of increased meal frequency. *New England Journal of Medicine* 321 (1989):929–934.

Leibowitz, S. Brain neurochemical systems controlling appetite and body weight gain. In *Obesity and Cachexia,* N.J. Rothwell and M.J. Stock, eds. New York: Wiley, 1991. A comprehensive summary of evidence supporting a role for brain neurochemical systems in the control of eating behavior and body weight.

Leibowitz, S. Neurochemical-neuroendocrine systems in the brain controlling macronutrient intake and metabolism. *Trends in Neurosciences* 15(12) (1992):491–497.

Leibowitz, S., and T. Kim. Impact of a galanin antagonist on exogenous galanin and natural patterns of fat ingestion. *Brain Research* 599 (1992):148–152.

Rolls, B.J. Carbohydrates, fats, and satiety. *American Journal of Clinical Nutrition* 61 (suppl. 1995):980S–987S.

Rolls, B. Determinants of food intale and selection. In *Nutrition in the 90's: Current Controversies and Analysis,* eds. G.E. Gaull, F.N. Kotsonis, and M.A. Mackey. New York: Marcel Dekker, Inc., 1990.

Rolls, B.J., et al. *Changing Hedonic Responses to Foods during and after a Meal.* New York: Academic Press, 1986.

Rolls, B.J., et al. Foods with different satiating effects in humans. *Appetite* 15 (1990):115–126.

Stubbs, R.J. Macronutrients, appetite and energy balance in humans. 1993 Ph.D. thesis. Cambridge University, England.

Stubbs, R.J., G.R. Goldberg, P.R. Murgatroyd, and A.M. Prentice. Carbohydrate balance and day-to-day food intake in man. *American Journal of Clinical Nutrition* 57 (1993):897–903.

Stubbs, R.J., and C.G. Habron. Isoenergetic substitution of MCT for LCT: Effect on energy intake in ad libitum feeding man. *International Journal of Obesity* 19 Suppl. 2 (1995), P28 (abstract).

Stubbs, R.J., P. Ritz, W.A. Coward, and A.M. Prentice. The effect of covert manipulation of the dietary fat and energy density on food intake and substrate flux in ad libitum feeding men. *American Journal of Clinical Nutrition* 62 (1995):675–690.

Tremblay, A., et al. Alcohol and a high-fat diet: a combination favoring overfeeding. *American Journal of Clinical Nutrition* 62 (1995): 639–644.

Chapter 6: Drop Your Glucose Load

Abate, N., A. Garg, R.M. Pershock, J. Stray-Gundreson, and S.M. Grundy. Relationships of generalized and regional adiposity of insulin sensitivity in men. *Journal of Clinical Investigation.* Vol. 96 (July 1995).

Brand Miller, J. The importance of glycemic index in diabetes. *American Journal of Clinical Nutrition* 59 (suppl) (1994): 747S–752S.

Food Fats and Oils. Washington, D.C.: Institute of Shortening and Edible Oils, 1994.

Foster-Powell, K., and J. Brand Miller. International tables of glycemic index. *American Journal of Clinical Nutrition* 62 (1995): 871–935.

Jenkins, D.J.A., et al. The glycaemic index of foods tested in diabetic patients: A new basis for carbohydrate exchange favouring the use of legumes. *Diabetologia* 24 (1983):257–264.

Jenkins, D.J.A., et al. Rate of digestion of foods and postprandial glycaemia in normal and diabetic subjects. *British Medical Journal* 2 (1980):14–17.

Jenkins, D.J.A., T.M.S. Wolever, R.H. Taylor, et al. Glycemic index of foods: a physiological basis for carbohydrate exchange. *American Journal of Clinical Nutrition* 34 (1981):362–366.

Lean, M.E.J., T.S. Han, C.E. Morrison. Waist circumference as a measure for indicating need for weight management. *British Medical Journal* 311 (1995):158–161.

Saleron, J., et al. Dietary fiber, glycemic load, and risk of non-insulin-dependent diabetes mellitus in women. *Journal of the American Medical Association* 277(6) (1997):472–577.

Westphal, S.A., M.C. Gannon, and F.Q. Nuttall. Metabolic response to glucose ingested with various amounts of protein. *American Journal of Clinical Nutrition* 52 (1990):267–272.

Wolevar, T.M.S., et al. Glycaemic index of fruits and fruit products in patients with diabetes. *International Journal of Food Sciences and Nutrition* 43 (1993):205–212.

Wolevar, T.M.S., et al. Glycaemic index of 102 complex carbohydrate foods in patients and diabetes. *Nutrition Research* 14 (5) (1994):651–669.

Wolever, T.M.S., and D.J.A. Jenkins. The use of the glycemic index in predicting the blood glucose response to mixed meals. *American Journal of Clinical Nutrition* 43 (1986):167–172.

Chapter 7: Hard Foods, Hard Bodies

Abate, N., et al. Relationships of generalized and regional adiposity to insulin sensitivity in men. *Journal of Clinical Investigation,* vol. 96 (1995).

Behall, K.M., et al. Diets containing high amylose vs. amylopectin starch: Effects on metabolic variables in human subjects. *American Journal of Clinical Nutrition* 49 (1989):337–43.

Behall, K.M. Effect of starch structure on glucose and insulin response in adults. *American Journal of Clinical Nutrition* 177 (1988): 128–132.

Brand Miller, J., et al. Rice: a high or low glycemic index food? *American Journal of Clinical Nutrition* 56 (1992):1034–1037.

Kuczmarski, R.J., et al. Increasing prevalence of overweight among US adults: The national health and nutrition examination surveys, 1960 to 1991. *Journal of the American Medical Association* 272 (1994):205–211.

Manson, J.E., et al. Body weight and mortality among women. *New England Journal of Medicine* 333 (1995):677–685.

Montignac, Michel. *Dine Out and Lose Weight*. Montignac USA, Inc., 1995.

Pi-Sunyer, F.X. Health implications of obesity. *American Journal of Clinical Nutrition* 53 (1991):1595S–1603S.

Pi-Sunyer, F.X. Medical hazards of obesity. *American Journal of Clinical Nutrition* 55 (1993): 655–660.

Troiano, R.P., Overweight prevalence and trends for children and adolescents. *Archives of Pediatric and Adolescent Medicine* 149 (1995): 1085–1091.

Welsh, S.O., and R.R.M. Marston. Review of trends in food use in the United States, 1909 to 1980. *Journal of the American Dietetic Association* 81 (1982):120–125.

Chapter 8: Protein

Ash, J., and S. Goldstein. *American Game Cooking*. Boston: Addison Wesley, 1991.

Chemical and Nutritional Composition of Fishes, Whales, Crustaceans, Mollusks and Their Products. Sidwell. NOAA Technical Memorandum MMFS F/SEC-11, US Department of Commerce, 1981.

Composition of Foods: Finfish and Shellfish Products. US Department of Commerce, 1981. USDA Handbook Eight. (Revised 1987).

Drew, K.R. Venison and other deer products. *North American Deer Farmer*, Spring 1995.

Eaton, S.B., and M. Konner. Paleolithic nutrition: a consideration of its nature and current implications. *New England Journal of Medicine* 312 (1985):283–289.

Recommended Dietary Allowances, Revised 1989. Food and Nutrition Board National Academy of Sciences—National Research

Council, Washington, D.C. USDA Human Nutrition Information Service Agriculture Handbook #8. Revised Dec. 1986.

Wang Y.J., et al. Omega-3 fatty acids in Lake Superior fish. *Journal of Food Science* 55 (1990):71–73.

Chapter 9: Hard Fibers

Anderson, J.W. *Plant Foods and Fiber.* HCF Nutrition Research Foundation, Inc., 1990.

Anderson, J.W., et al. Postprandial serum glucose, insulin, and lipoprotein responses to high- and low-fiber diets. *Metabolism* 44 (1955):848–854.

Anderson, J.W., et al. Dietary fiber and diabetes: A comprehensive review and practical application. *Journal of the American Dietetic Association.* 87 (1987):1189–1198.

Anderson, J.W., and S.R. Bridges. Dietary fiber content of selected foods. *American Journal of Clinical Nutrition* 47 (1988):440–447.

Anderson, J.W., and C.A. Bryant. Dietry fiber: diabetes and obesity. *American Journal of Gastroenterology* 81 (1986):898–906.

Anderson, J.W., B.M. Smith, and N.J. Gustafson. Health benefits and practical aspects of high-fiber diets. *American Journal of Clinical Nutrition* 59 (1994):1242S–1247S.

Anderson, J.W., and K. Ward. High-carbohydrate high fiber diets for insulin-treated men with diabetes mellitus. *American Journal of Clinical Nutrition* 32 (1979):2312–2321.

Blackburn, N.A., et al. The mechanism of action of guar gum in improving glucose tolerance in man. *Clinical Science* 66 (1984): 329.

Geil, P.B., and J.W. Anderson. Health benefits of dietary fiber. *Medical Exercise, Nutrition and Health* 1 (1992):257–271.

Greenwald, P., et al. Dietary fiber in the reduction of colon cancer risk. *Journal of the American Dietetic Association* 87 (1987): 1178–1188.

Jenkins, D.J.A., et al. Fiber and starchy food: Gut function and implications in disease. *American Journal of Gastroenterology* 81 (1986): 920–930.

Klurfeld, D.M. The role of dietary fiber in gastrointestinal disease. *Journal of the American Dietetic Association* 87 (1987):1172–1177.

Rimm, E.R., et al. Vegetable, fruit, and cereal fiber intake and risk of coronary heart disease among men. *Journal of the American Medical Association* 275 (1996):447–451.

Trowell, H. Obesity in Western World. *Plant Foods Man* 1 (1975): 157.

Chapter 10: Hard Beans

Anderson, J.W. *Plant Foods and Fiber.* HCF Nutrition Research Foundation, Inc., 1990.

Anderson, J.W., et al. Meta-analysis of the effects of soy protein intake on serum lipids. *New England Journal of Medicine* 333 (1995): 276–282.

Carroll K., and E.M. Kurowska. Soy consumption and cholesterol reduction: review of animal and human studies. *Journal of Nutrition* 125 (1995):594S–597S.

Foster-Powell, K., and J. Brand Miller. International tables of glycemic index. *American Journal of Clinical Nutrition* 62 (1995): 871S–893S.

Geil, P.B., and J.W. Anderson. Dry beans: a review of nutrition and health implications. *Journal of the American College of Nutrition.* In press.

Kelin, B.P. Potential public health impact of soy protein: incorporating soy proteins into baked products for use in clincial studies. *Journal of Nutrition* 125 (1995):666S–674S.

Leathwood, P., and P. Pollet. Effects of slow release carbohydrates in the form of bean flakes on the evolution of hunger and satiety in man. *Appetite* 10 (1988):1.

Messina, M., and J.J.W. Erdman Jr., eds. First internation symposium on the role of soy in preventing and treating chronic disease. *Journal of Nutrition* 125 (1995):567S–808S.

Weber, C.W. *Traditional Desert Foods Fiber Content Analysis Chart.* Native Seeds/SEARCH, 1991.

Chapter 11: Hard Grains

Anderson, J.W. *Plant Foods and Fiber.* HCF Nutrition Research Foundation, Inc., 1990.

Foster-Powell, K., and J. Brand Miller. International tables of glycemic index. *American Journal of Clinical Nutrition* 62 (1995): 871S–893S.

Hallfrisch, J., et al. Diets containing soluble oat extracts improve glucose insulin responses of moderately hypercholesteroemic men and women. *American Journal of Clinical Nutrition* 61(1995):379–384.

Chapter 12: Beans and Grains

Anderson, J.W. *Plant Foods and Fiber.* HCF Nutrition Research Foundation, Inc., 1990.

Foster-Powell, K., and J. Brand Miller. International tables of glycemic index. *American Journal of Clinical Nutrition* 62 (1995): 871S–893S.

Chapter 13: Hard Veggies

Anderson, J.W. *Plant Foods and Fiber.* HCF Nutrition Research Foundation, Inc., 1990.

Foster-Powell, K., and J. Brand Miller. International tables of glycemic index. *American Journal of Clinical Nutrition* 62 (1995): 871S–893S.

Chapter 14: Hard Fruits

Anderson, J.W. *Plant Foods and Fiber.* HCF Nutrition Research Foundation, Inc., 1990.

Foster-Powell, K., and J. Brand Miller. International tables of glycemic index. *American Journal of Clinical Nutrition* 62 (1995): 871S–893S.

Chapter 17: Hard Cuisine

Campbell, T.C. Meat—can we live without it? Diet, nutrition and the prevention of chronic diseases. *World Health Forum* 12 (1991):251–283.

Campbell, T.C., et al. Diets and cancer mortality rates in sixty-five counties in the People's Republic of China. Pennington Biomedical Research Center Reports, 1992, pp. 130–143.

Chen, J., et al. The change of disease patterns and control strategies. *Chinese Journal of Preventive Medicine* 4 (1990):291–293.

Chen, J., T.C. Campbell, J. Li, and R. Peto. *Diet, Life-style and Mortality in China. A Study of the Characteristics of 65 Chinese Counties.* Oxford: Oxford University Press; Ithaca, NY: Cornell University Press; Beijing: People's Medical Publishing House, 1991.

Ferro-Luzzi, A., and F. Branca. Mediterranean diet, Italian-style: prototype of a healthy diet. *American Journal of Clinical Nutrition* 61 (1995):1338S–1345S.

Helsing, E. Traditional diets and disease patterns of the Mediterranean, circa 1960. *American Journal of Clinical Nutrition* 61(1995): 1329S–1337S.

Hu, J., et al. Dietary calcium and bone density among middle-aged and elderly women in China. *American Journal of Clinical Nutrition* 58 (1993):219–227.

James, W.P.T. Nutrition science and policy research: implications for Mediterranean diets. *American Journal of Clinical Nutrition* 61 (1995):132–8S.

Kafatos, A., et al. Coronary heart disease risk-factor status of the Cretan urban population in the 1980's. *American Journal of Clinical Nutrition* 54 (1991):591–598.

Keys, A. Mediterranean diet and public health: personal reflections. *American Journal of Clinical Nutrition* 61(1995):1321S–1323S.

Keys, A. *Seven Countries: A Multivariate Analysis of Death and Coronary Heart Disease.* Cambridge, MA: Harvard University Press, 1980.

Nestle, M. Mediteranean diets: historical and research overview. *American Journal of Clinical Nutrition* 61 (1995):113S–120S.

Parpia, B. Socioeconomic determinants of food and nutrient intakes in rural China. Ph.D. Dissertation. Cornell University, Ithaca, NY, 1994.

Renaud, S. Cretan Mediterranean diet for prevention of coronary heart disease. *American Journal of Clinical Nutrition* 61 (1995): 1360S–1367S.

Tavani, A. Fruit and vegetable consumption and cancer risk in a Mediterranean population. *American Journal of Clinical Nutrition* 61 (1995):1374S–1377S.

Trichopoulou, A., et al. Diet and survival of elderly Greeks: a link to the past. *American Journal of Clinical Nutrition* 61 (1995):1346S–50S.

Wang, G., et al. Dietary fiber composition of selected foods in the People's Republic of China. *Journal of Food Composition* 4 (1991):293–303.

Willett, W.C. Diet and health: What should we eat? *Science* 264 (1994):532–537.

Willett, W.C. Mediterranean diet pyramid: a cultural model for healthy eating. *American Journal of Clinical Nutrition* 61 (1995): 1402S–1406S.

Chapter 18: Fat-Ripping Exercises

Ainsworth, B.E., et al. Compendium of physical activities: classification of energy costs of human physical activities. *Medicine and Science in Sports and Exercise* 25 (1993):71–80.

Barnard, R.J., et al. Diet, not aging causes skeletal muscle insulin resistance. *Gerontology* 41 (1995):205–211.

Barnard, R.J. Exercise and diet in the prevention and control of the metabolic syndrome. *Sports Medicine* 18 (1994):218–228.

Leibel, R.L., et al. Changes in energy expenditure resulting from altered body weight. *New England Journal of Medicine* 332 (1995): 621–628.

Romieu, I., et al. Energy intake and other determinants of relative weight. *American Journal of Clinical Nutrition* 47 (1988):406–412.

Zeni, A.I. Energy expenditure with indoor exercise machines. *Journal of the American Medical Association* 275 (1996):1424–1427.

Chapter 19: Building a Fat-Burning Engine

Fleck, S.J., and W.J. Kraemer. *Designing Resistance Training Programs.* Human Kinetics Books, 1987.

Schwarzenegger, A. *Arnold Schwarzenegger's Encyclopedia of Modern Bodybuilding.* New York: Simon & Schuster, 1985.

Chapter 20: The Glucose Epidemic

Boyce, V.L., and B.A. Swinburn. The traditional Pima Indian diet. Composition and adaption for use in a dietary intervention study. *Diabetes Care* 16 (1993):369–371.

Brand, J.C., et al. Plasma glucose and insulin responses to traditional Pima Indian meals. *American Journal of Clinical Nutrition* 51 (1990):416–420.

Fernandez, M.L., et al. Pectin isolated from prickly pear modifies low density lipoprotein metabolism in cholesterol-fed guinea pigs. *Journal of Nutrition* 120 (1990):1283–1290.

Knowler, W.C., et al. Diabetes incidence in Pima Indians contributions of obesity and parental diabetes. *American Journal of Epidemiology* 113 (1981):144–156.

Nabhan, G.P. Food health and native American agriculture. In *Our Sustainable Table,* R. Clark, ed. San Francisco: North Point Press, 1990.

O'Dea, K. Marked improvement in carbohydrate and lipid metabolism in diabetic australian aborigines after temporary reversion to traditional lifestyle. *Diabetes* 33 (1984):596–602.

Winkelman, M. *Journal of Pharmacological Properties of Some Piman (O'Odham) Medicinal Plants for the Treatment of Diabetes.* Native Seeds/SEARCH Monograph No. 1.